9 HABITS

OF HAPPY RETIREES

Discover the Secrets to a Fulfilling Retirement

Sarah Barry

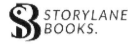
STORYLANE
BOOKS.

Published by

Storylane Books

hello@storylanebooks.com

www.storylanebooks.com

TABLE OF CONTENTS

INTRODUCTION

Retirement offers the opportunity to shape each day into a masterpiece of joy, fulfillment, and adventure. No longer bound by the constraints of a work schedule, every day becomes a canvas awaiting your vibrant strokes of color.

Before starting this exciting journey, let's take a moment to set the stage. Due to a change in the population where older people are expected to outnumber younger ones sooner than expected, it's crucial that we rethink what retirement means.

Financial planning is important, but let's be real—retirement isn't just about padding your nest egg. It's about embracing a lifestyle that brings you genuine happiness and fulfillment. That's where this book comes in.

In the pages ahead, we'll travel a path together, discovering the nine habits of happy retirees. We will start by moving through the different phases of retirement, talk about how to cultivate a positive mindset, just how to leave a lasting legacy, tips for travel and adventure, and so much more.

Picture it: you, basking in the glow of a life well-lived, surrounded by laughter, love, and endless possibilities. Sound too good to be true? Think again! With plenty of humor, a hefty dose of wisdom, and loads of practical advice, you can pave the way for retirement dreams worth living.

So, what can you expect between these pages? Well let's take a closer look:

- Embracing a modern approach to retirement planning.

- Understanding retirement and how to thrive within it.

- Fostering a mindset that breeds joy and contentment in retirement.

- Exploring passions and hobbies to keep life exciting and fulfilling.

- Staying active and healthy to make the most of your retirement adventures.

- Nurturing relationships with friends, family, and peers for a rich retirement experience.

- Keeping your mind sharp and engaged through continuous learning and personal growth.

- Finding purpose and fulfillment through volunteering and philanthropy.

- Seizing the opportunity for adventure and exploration in retirement.

I offer you the chance to imagine the retirement you've always dreamed of. I encourage you to stop, take a deep breath, and commit to actively starting the process of turning that dream into a reality.

Start by asking yourself:

- How do you envision your ideal retirement lifestyle, and does it align with your values, interests, and priorities?

- What strategies do you have in place for coping with the emotional aspects of retirement, such as adjusting to a new routine, finding meaning and fulfillment, or combating feelings of loneliness or isolation?

- What legacy do you hope to leave behind in retirement, whether it's through charitable giving, mentoring future generations, or pursuing personal passions?

Not sure of the answers? Don't worry; the goal of this book is to help you explore the answers and map out a fulfilling, empowering, and positive retirement. Are you ready to get started?

CHAPTER 1:
PREPARING FOR RETIREMENT
ON A WHOLE NEW LEVEL

For too long, retirement planning has been synonymous with financial planning. Having a comfortable nest egg is essential, but what good is it if you haven't considered how you will fill your days once the alarm clock is retired too?

In these pages, we will explore the often-overlooked aspects of retirement planning. The content will take a look at why your post-career satisfaction is directly tied to how you manage your newfound freedom.

Retirement is not a one-size-fits-all affair. Gone are the days when retirement meant settling into a rocking chair with a knitting needle or a pipe. Today, retirees are a vibrant, diverse bunch, spanning a spectrum of interests, passions, and energy levels.

Whether you dream of traveling the world, finally mastering salsa dancing, starting a new business venture, or simply spending more time with loved ones, this chapter serves as your roadmap to making the most of your retirement years. It's about crafting a life that is fulfilling, purposeful, and wonderfully yours.

The Impact of Retirement on Mental and Emotional Well-Being

Imagine this: You have saved up all your life, got your retirement fund sorted, and are ready to kick back and enjoy the good life. But suddenly, you find yourself feeling a bit... off. Perhaps you're feeling lonely or struggling to find your sense of purpose now that you're not punching the clock every day.

Many retirees find themselves grappling with issues like:

- **Loss of identity:** For many retirees, your job may have been a significant part of your identity. When you retire, you might struggle with feelings of loss and uncertainty about who you are now that you're no longer working.

- **Social isolation:** You might find yourself spending less time around coworkers and friends you used to see regularly. This can lead to feelings of loneliness and isolation, especially if you don't have a strong support network outside of work.

- **Lack of purpose:** Without the structure of a job, you might struggle to find meaning and purpose in your daily life. You might feel adrift, unsure of what to do with your time or how to fill your days.

- **Financial stress:** Even if you have saved diligently for retirement, you may still worry about your financial security. You might fear running out of money or not being able to afford unexpected expenses, which can lead to stress and anxiety.

- **Health concerns:** As you age, you may experience declining health or chronic health conditions. Dealing with health issues can take a toll on your mental well-being and lead to feelings of frustration, sadness, or anxiety.

- **Family dynamics:** Retirement can change the dynamics of family relationships, especially if you find yourself spending more time with your spouse or adult children. Conflicts or tensions within the family can contribute to stress and emotional strain.

- **Boredom:** With all the free time that retirement brings, some may struggle to stay engaged and stimulated. Boredom can lead to feelings of restlessness or dissatisfaction with life.

- **Existential concerns:** Retirement can prompt you to reflect on your life and confront existential questions about purpose, mortality, and the meaning of life. These deep, philosophical issues can be challenging to grapple with and may cause emotional distress.

These challenges highlight the importance of prioritizing mental and emotional well-being in retirement planning. By acknowledging and addressing these issues, you can take proactive steps to maintain a fulfilling and satisfying quality of life during this next phase of life.

Financial stability is crucial, but it's only part of the puzzle. True wealth goes beyond dollars and cents. It's about having enough time, energy, love, and meaningful connections to fill your days with joy and fulfillment.

That's why it's essential to think beyond the bank balance when planning for retirement. Ask yourself: What activities bring me joy? How can I stay connected with others? What kind of legacy do I want to leave behind?

It's about crafting a lifestyle that lights you up from the inside out. The key is to stay engaged and connected with the world around you.

Be mindful and continue to check in with yourself from time to time. If you're feeling down or overwhelmed, don't be afraid to reach out for support. Whether talking to a friend, joining a support group, or seeking professional help, there's no shame in asking for a helping hand.

The Importance of Planning

Retirement is a bit like starting a new book, and just like any good story, it's more satisfying when you have a sense of direction.

So, grab a pen and paper or your favorite planning app, and start brainstorming. What are some things you've always wanted to do but never had the time for? Maybe it's learning a new skill, traveling to a dream destination, volunteering for a cause you're passionate about, or finally tackling that home improvement project you've been putting off. The possibilities are endless!

But here's the thing: It's not just about keeping busy. It's about finding activities that really fill your cup and give you a sense of purpose. That brings us to the second part of the equation: finding meaningful activities.

Now, what do I mean by "meaningful activities"? Simply put, these are the things that put a smile on your face and make you feel like a great person. They're the activities that make you feel like you're making a difference, whether in your own life or the lives of others. It could be joining a book club, where you can connect with other avid readers and engage in stimulating discussions. Or maybe it's taking up gardening and reveling in the satisfaction of watching your plants thrive under your care.

The key here is to tap into your passions and interests. What gets you excited? What makes you feel alive? Don't be afraid to try new things and step outside your comfort zone. Retirement is the perfect time to explore, experiment, and discover new passions.

Coping Strategies

Retirement is like stepping into a whole new world, and sometimes, it can feel like you're navigating without a map. I would like to share some strategies that can help you keep your mental health in tip-top shape.

- **Embrace the change:** Acknowledge that it's okay to feel a mix of emotions. Retirement is a big change, and it's natural to feel a bit unsettled at first. Give yourself permission to feel whatever comes up, whether it's excitement, uncertainty, or even a touch of sadness for leaving your old routine behind.

- **Stay connected:** One of the biggest challenges you will face is a shift in social dynamics. Suddenly, your daily interactions at the office might be replaced with more solitary time. Combat loneliness by staying connected with friends, family, and your community. Social connections can be a lifeline for our mental well-being.

- **Get involved:** Find new passions and activities that bring you joy and fulfillment. This is a great way to give your life purpose and meaning.

- **Establish a routine:** While retirement might mean saying goodbye to the daily grind, it doesn't mean throwing structure out the window altogether. Establishing a daily routine can provide a sense of stability and purpose. It doesn't have to be rigid; think of it more like a loose framework to guide your days and keep you feeling productive.

- **Move your body:** Physical activity isn't just good for your body—it's also a powerful mood booster. Make time for regular exercise, whether it's going for walks, hitting the gym, or practicing yoga. Not only will it keep you healthy and energized, but it can also help alleviate stress and improve your mood.

- **Practice gratitude:** Take a moment each day to reflect on the things you're grateful for. It's easy to get caught up in what's missing or what you wish you had, but focusing on the positives can shift your perspective and foster a greater sense of contentment.

- **Ask for help:** If you struggle with overwhelming emotions or are persistently down, don't hesitate to seek professional support. Talking to a therapist or counselor can provide you with valuable tools and strategies for managing your mental health during this transition.

Embrace the ups and downs, and don't be afraid to lean on your support system when you need it. With the right mindset and a little bit of self-care, you can navigate this new chapter with confidence and joy.

The Connection Between Time Management and Post-Career Satisfaction

Mastering time management isn't about squeezing your newfound freedom into a rigid schedule. It's about crafting a retirement that's as fulfilling as it is fun.

So, here you are, finally retired, and the world is your oyster. No more pesky alarm clocks, no more rushing to beat the morning traffic. It's all about sleeping in, indulging in your favorite hobbies, and kicking back without a care in the world. Sounds dreamy, right? Well, it can be—for a little while.

But here's the issue: Without some semblance of structure, those blissful days can quickly turn into a blur of Netflix binges and endless scrolling. Before you know it, you're stuck in a rut of routine, wondering where all the time went.

That's when you can put effective time management into practice. Now, I'm not talking about micromanaging every minute of our day. Instead, it's about finding a balance that works—one that lets you pursue your passions while still leaving room for spontaneity.

How do you achieve that ideal equilibrium? Well, it all starts with knowing what floats your boat. What motivates you to get out of bed in the morning? Whether it's painting, golf, or catching up with friends, you need to jot them down and make them a priority.

Next up, it's time to get organized. You can go old-school with a trusty day planner or embrace the digital age with apps like Trello or Google Calendar. The choice is yours, so pick whatever you feel comfortable with.

Now, please remember that consistency is key. If you want to be serious about finally writing that novel or perfecting your golf swing, you need to carve out time for it every day. Those small chunks of time add up, even if it's just 15 minutes.

Of course, don't forget to leave room for life's little surprises. Retirement is all about flexibility, so it's okay if you stray from the plan every now and then. Embrace the spontaneity, and remember that it's all part of the adventure.

Let's talk about downtime. It's important to give yourself permission to kick back and relax guilt-free. Whether it's going to the movies or losing yourself in a good book, make time for the things that recharge your batteries.

You need to remember that time is precious. And in retirement, it's more finite than ever. So you need to make every moment count. Whether you're ticking off your bucket list or simply savoring the little things, remember to live with purpose, passion, and plenty of pizzazz.

Strategies for Cultivating Retirement Happiness

Once you've established a retirement plan, it's crucial to prioritize those parts of life that money can't buy. Here are some positive strategies that research indicates can enhance life fulfillment during retirement:

- **Focus on maintaining good health:** It all boils down to, "What good is money if you can't enjoy it?" Money's value lies in enjoyment. Retirees prioritize good health for a happy retirement. Exercise and a healthy diet lower health risks, boost energy, strengthen immunity, and enhance mood (*Never Too Late*, 2011).

  - **Tips:** It's never too late to start getting active and eating good stuff! Studies reveal that even late bloomers who kickstart their fitness journey and embrace a nutritious diet can significantly slash the chances of heart problems and outlive their buddies. It is suggested that we aim for 150 to 300 minutes of moderate exercise weekly (*Never Too Late*, 2011).

- **Nurture social connections:** Want to boost your happiness in retirement? Enjoy hobbies with loved ones! Research shows that socializing more can lead to a happier life. On the flip side, being socially isolated can be as bad for your health as smoking, obesity, or not exercising (Crabtree, 2011). So, keep those social connections strong for a healthier, happier you!

  - **Tips:** You can keep in touch by joining fun social events at your community center or library. Think game nights, movie outings, museum trips, and book clubs. Zoom and Google Hangouts are perfect for video calls, and you can even have virtual movie nights with friends afar using Netflix Party.

- **Train to be optimistic:** Having a sunny disposition isn't just good for the soul; it's a lifesaver! Research shows that optimists have healthier hearts, live longer, and dodge chronic illnesses. In fact, optimists are less likely to have heart attacks and more likely to reach a ripe old age (Lee et al., 2019).

- o **Tips:** Believe it or not, becoming an optimist is totally doable! Research proves that you can train your brain to see the bright side of things by doing easy exercises. It's like giving your brain a positivity makeover! And remember, hang out with sunny-minded people and maybe take a news break to keep the good vibes flowing (Lee et al., 2019)!

- **Try owning a pet:** Rover isn't just about cuddles; he's your ticket to a more active lifestyle! Research shows that older dog owners who walk their furry friends daily are 20% more active than those without dogs and spend 30 fewer minutes being inactive each day (Wu et al., 2017). If a dog isn't your style, consider low-maintenance pals like cats and birds!

  - o **Tips:** Having a furry companion can be just as rewarding as having a human buddy. To find your next four-legged friend, visit your local animal shelter. If you're not ready for full-time dog ownership, consider becoming a foster parent. You can provide temporary care for a dog from a rescue center for a few days, weeks, or even longer, helping them find a loving home. If this is too much, remember you can volunteer at an animal shelter as well. Remember, all dogs are great, regardless of their size!

- **Learning for a lifetime:** Retirement is about embracing new experiences and continuing to grow intellectually. Curiosity is the key to lifelong learning, which doesn't have to be formal or structured. It's about keeping your mind active and engaged, no matter what form that takes. So, keep never stop seeking knowledge!

  - o **Tips:** Many communities offer classes, workshops, and seminars specifically geared toward retirees. Take advantage of these opportunities to learn from experts and connect with like-minded individuals.

- **Exploring and adventure:** This is the perfect time to satisfy your wanderlust and embrace new travel experiences. Traveling doesn't have to mean jetting off to exotic destinations. It could be as simple as taking a road trip to a nearby town you've never visited or exploring a local hiking trail. The key is to keep exploring and discovering new places.

- o **Tips:** Be open to new experiences and opportunities that come your way. Say yes to invitations, even if they push you out of your comfort zone. You never know what adventures await when you embrace new possibilities. Remember, adventure is a mindset as much as it is an activity. Approach life with a sense of curiosity and wonder, and you'll find that adventure is always just around the corner.

- **Giving back:** Retirement is a time to reflect on the blessings in your life and find ways to give back to others. Volunteering is a wonderful way to give back to your community and make a positive impact. Whether it's serving meals at a soup kitchen, tutoring children, or helping out at a local animal shelter, there are countless ways to volunteer your time and talents.

- o **Tips:** Remember, giving back isn't just about making a difference in the lives of others—it's also about finding fulfillment and purpose in your own life. By giving back, you'll not only make the world a better place, but you'll also enrich your own retirement experience in ways you never imagined.

Overcoming Common Misconceptions About Retirement

Many misconceptions surround retirement. Unfortunately, most retirees aren't aware of them until they are actually retired. Let's address some of those now:

- **Misconception #1: Retirement is just a 30-year vacation:** If only it were that simple. Sure, lounging on a beach sounds dreamy, but studies show that too much downtime can actually lead to the blues. It turns out that staying active and engaged is the real ticket to happiness (*Five Common Misconceptions*, 2023).

And hey, if you want to keep working, go for it! Voluntary part-timers are the happiest campers around.

- **Misconception #2: It's all about the Benjamins:** Money is undoubtedly important; however, good health takes precedence over financial wealth. Interestingly, you don't need immense wealth to savor retirement. As long as there is enough to meet the essential needs, you can lead a fulfilling life post-retirement.

- **Misconception #3: Spending stays steady:** Retirement spending resembles a rollercoaster rather than a lazy river. Initially, you might indulge in travel expenses, but over time, these expenses change. Rising health care costs and unexpected family obligations emerge—all important factors to consider.

- **Misconception #4: It's a two-player game:** Retirement is not exclusive to couples. Whether you are on your own or with a companion, it's all about being true to yourself. Additionally, women typically outlive men by an average of six years. Therefore, it's important to celebrate your independence and take charge of your retirement path.

- **Misconception #5: Financial planning ends at retirement:** Retirement marks the end of your career, yet it signals the start of a fresh chapter. There is still a lot of planning ahead, from estate affairs to healthcare necessities. Stay sharp, stay savvy, and keep those financial gears turning!

- **Misconception #6: Retirement's all about relaxing:** Retirement is your chance to shine, to chase after those dreams you've been putting on hold. It's about doing, not just being done. So, what's your retirement vision? Get clear on those goals and start making moves!

- **Misconception #7: You have to punch out at a certain age:** Retirement age is just a number. If you love what you do, why hang up your hat? Work can be fulfilling in so many ways—socially, mentally, emotionally. And if you do decide to retire, take your time transitioning. Building a new community and finding new passions doesn't happen overnight.

- **Misconception #8: Retirement is a universal experience:** There was a time, likely when your parents retired, when it looked the same for most. You finished your last day of work and were expected to spend your days, well, doing nothing. The thought process was that you earned this time to rest and relax. Now, retirement is as diverse as those entering this exciting phase of life. Today's retirees are rewriting the script, embracing new opportunities, and living life to the fullest. Retirees view this phase as a chance to redefine themselves, explore new passions, and make the most of their time.

Life moves fast, taking everything along with it, including retirement. The changing retirement landscape continues to lead to a variety of misconceptions. Just be mindful that your retirement journey is just that, yours! Make it uniquely you.

Okay, let's take a moment to reflect on what we've just covered. We've tossed aside the outdated notions of retirement being just about financial planning. Instead, we've explored the deeper layers of what it means to retire with gusto and purpose.

As we turn the page on this chapter, I want you to get excited. Why? Because we're about to dive headfirst into the world of navigating the different phases of retirement.

From the initial exhilaration of newfound freedom to the occasional twinges of uncertainty, each phase brings its own set of joys and challenges. It is time to discover strategies to tackle all of them and gain the confidence we deserve.

CHAPTER 2:
NAVIGATING THE DIFFERENT PHASES
OF RETIREMENT

In this chapter, we will explore the dynamic evolution of retirement. Retirement is no longer about simply relaxing in a rocking chair and observing life pass by. Today's retirees are redefining retirement norms, seeking new experiences, and creating meaningful impacts.

We will begin by exploring the transition phase, which is the period when you adjust to the routines of your previous life and navigate your way through this new chapter.

Next up, we'll tackle the phases of retirement head-on. From the honeymoon phase, where you're basking in the glow of newfound freedom, to the disillusionment phase, where reality hits and you realize retirement isn't quite what you expected.

And finally, we'll explore the legacy stage. Because retirement isn't just about living your best life in the present; it's also about creating a lasting impact for future generations. Whether it's through mentoring, volunteering, or simply sharing your wisdom, there are endless ways to leave your mark on the world.

The Pre-Retirement Phase

So, retirement is more than just leaving work for the last time and relaxing into the sunset with a piña colada in hand (although that does sound pretty great). It's a complete journey, filled with unexpected twists, turns, and perhaps a few detours along the way.

Retirement has distinct phases. The initial one, known as the pre-retirement phase or the "planning party," marks the beginning of this next amazing part of your life.

During this phase, which can last anywhere from a few years to a decade (depending on how eager you are to hang up your badge), you're not just crunching numbers for your retirement fund. You're also mentally prepping for the big shift.

Picture a time when selecting your next vacation destination brings more joy than receiving a promotion. Welcome to the pre-retirement phase! It's just like the anticipation of New Year's Eve, except instead of celebrating with champagne, you're contemplating questions such as, "Where do I envision living?" and "Is it time to master salsa dancing?"

It's normal to feel a bit antsy during this time. You're straddling the line between excitement and uncertainty. Did you know that research shows that those who plan for their retirement tend to feel happier once they get there (Prvulovic, 2022)?

Now, let's discuss strategy. Here are the steps you can take to ensure the strength of your retirement plan:

- **Dream big:**
  - **Visualize your ideal retirement:** Take a moment to envision your perfect retirement scenario. Whether it's sipping cocktails on a tropical beach, pursuing creative passions, or embarking on epic adventures, let your imagination run wild.
  - **Write it down:** Grab a pen and paper (or open a digital notebook) and jot down your retirement dreams. Putting your aspirations into words solidifies them and sets the stage for turning them into reality.
  - **Make a plan:** Transform your dreams into actionable goals. Break down your aspirations into smaller steps and create a timeline for achieving them. Whether it's saving a specific amount of money, learning new skills, or researching travel destinations, every step brings you closer to your dream retirement.

- **Health is wealth:**

  - **Prioritize self-care:** Retirement is your time to shine, so prioritize your health and well-being. Start by adopting healthier habits such as eating nutritious foods, staying active through regular exercise, and getting sufficient rest.

  - **Stay proactive with healthcare:** Schedule regular check-ups with your healthcare provider and stay proactive about managing any existing health conditions. Prevention and early intervention are key to maintaining optimal health throughout retirement.

  - **Embrace holistic wellness:** Focus on holistic wellness by nurturing your physical, mental, and emotional health. Incorporate activities that bring joy, reduce stress, and foster a sense of purpose into your daily routine.

- **Money matters:**

  - **Assess your financial situation:** Take a comprehensive look at your finances to ensure they're aligned with your retirement goals. Evaluate your savings, investments, and retirement accounts to determine if adjustments are needed.

  - **Develop a financial plan:** Create a solid financial plan that addresses your short-term and long-term financial needs. Consider factors such as budgeting, debt management, retirement income sources, and estate planning.

  - **Seek professional guidance:** If navigating finances feels overwhelming, don't hesitate to seek advice from financial advisors or retirement planners. They can provide personalized guidance and strategies to optimize your financial health for retirement.

- **Squad goals:**

  - **Cultivate meaningful relationships:** Retirement is an opportune time to strengthen existing connections and forge new friendships. Reach out to old friends, join clubs or interest groups, and participate in community activities to expand your social network.

- o **Nurture supportive relationships:** Surround yourself with supportive individuals who uplift and inspire you. Cultivate relationships that bring joy, laughter, and companionship into your life.

- o **Share experiences:** Embrace opportunities to share experiences and create memories with friends and loved ones. Whether it's traveling together, pursuing shared hobbies, or simply enjoying quality time, meaningful relationships enrich your retirement journey.

- **Timing is everything:**
  - o **Listen to your intuition:** Pay attention to your instincts and inner guidance when considering retirement timing. Reflect on your readiness for this significant life transition, and trust your intuition to guide you.

  - o **Consider practical factors:** Evaluate practical considerations such as financial readiness, healthcare needs, and personal fulfillment when determining the right time to retire. Assessing both emotional and logistical aspects ensures a smooth transition into retirement.

  - o **Plan strategically:** Take a strategic approach to retirement timing by considering factors such as market conditions, healthcare coverage, and lifestyle preferences. Balancing your desires with practical considerations sets the stage for a successful retirement journey.

By completing these tasks during this initial phase, you will pave the way for a retirement focused not only on relaxation but on embracing the best possible life. Prepare to celebrate, as your retirement years are poised to be truly exceptional!

The Honeymoon Phase

Welcome to the honeymoon phase, where life feels like a perpetual vacation, and the possibilities are as endless as the horizon.

Picture this: no more early morning rush hour, no more tight deadlines, and definitely no more annoying emails flooding your inbox. It's just you, your freedom, and a whole world waiting to be explored.

During this honeymoon stage, it's all about soaking up the bliss of newfound liberation. Embrace the change! Sure, it's normal to feel a tad uncertain amid this transition, but remember, you've got a lifetime of experience mastering challenges. This is simply another adventure waiting to happen.

Now, what to do with all this newfound freedom, you ask?

- **Embrace the transformation:** This period is a time of change, so feeling a bit uneasy is normal. Remember that you are meant to grow, learn, and overcome challenges in every stage of life. Focus on improving yourself and the new possibilities that retirement brings.

- **Establish a fresh routine:** Retirement is a great time to try new things and create healthy habits that match your interests and retirement plans.

- **Discover ways to remain physically engaged:** Engaging in activities such as going to the gym, trying new hobbies, or spending time outdoors can help you adjust to retirement by keeping your body and mind active.

Well, the world is full of opportunities for you to explore! Whether you are traveling to exotic destinations, experimenting with new hobbies, or simply indulging in some well-deserved relaxation, this is your moment to shine. Make the best of each opportunity that crosses your path. Make the most of every opportunity that comes your way.

Amidst all the fun and excitement, don't forget to think long-term. It's never too early to start crafting your retirement vision. What do you want the rest of your years to look like? What brings you joy and fulfillment?

When you are navigating a hectic schedule or savoring moments of tranquility, it is essential to discover what suits you best. Embrace the opportunities before you, seize the day, and ensure each moment is meaningful. This is your time to excel!

The Disenchantment Phase

Just as the initial excitement of a romantic honeymoon may diminish, the allure of retirement can also fade with time. While some may enjoy an extended period of post-retirement bliss that spans years, others might find themselves growing bored of retirement, experiencing a sense of stagnation rather than fulfillment.

In a 2022 survey, over half of retirees find their retirement lifestyle aligning with expectations. However, a whopping 21% rate their quality of life post-retirement as a letdown (Retirement Confidence Survey, 2022). Welcome to the disenchantment stage of retirement!

Feeling trapped in a monotonous retirement routine can be challenging. You may discover yourself engaging in tasks without a sense of purpose, resulting in restlessness and a lack of fulfillment.

It is important to know that you don't have to settle for a lackluster retirement. The biggest mistake retirees make? Following the crowd without stopping to think about what they actually want out of this chapter of life. It's time to chart your own course!

So, how can you break free from the disenchanted state? By dedicating time to introspection, rekindling connections with passions, and redefining the concept of success. Rest assured, discovering clarity and purpose in retirement can be transformative.

Now, let's talk strategy. During this tough phase, it's crucial to manage your expectations and be realistic about the phases of retirement. Don't just sit back and let retirement happen to you—take the reins and make it your own!

To prepare for success during the disenchantment stage and maximize your retirement years, try the following:

- **Have practical expectations:** Retirement is like a rollercoaster ride of life, so hold on tight and enjoy the unexpected twists and turns. Don't anticipate perfection in retirement; it's a journey filled with highs and lows and plenty of chances to bloom.

- **Take initiative and get help:** Don't sit around waiting for retirement to tap you on the shoulder. Seize the reins of your ideal life! Strategize in advance, seek advice from those with experience, and enlist the necessary support to master the art of maximizing your time and energy.

- **Establish personal goals for your life:** After the honeymoon phase fades, it's time to shift focus to something meaningful. Retirement offers the chance to tackle those long-awaited tasks and delve into new adventures.

Be patient and continue exploring until you discover what resonates with you. Always strive for personal growth.

Reorientation Phases

So, you have now moved through the challenging phase—the disenchantment period. It's the moment when you come to the realization that retirement differs from its portrayal in movies. Did you miss that sense of purpose? Don't worry, this is a common experience.

Now, it's time to rebuild. Think of it as a do-it-yourself project for your identity and lifestyle. It's about finding what gets your heart racing and what makes you excited for life once again.

This phase focuses on embracing change and shaking things up. Wishing for the past won't bring it back, so it's time to craft a new version of yourself in retirement. Grab your toolbox, and let's start re-orienting!

After years of balancing various roles, retirement presents a golden opportunity to look into your true self (the unfiltered version) and determine what truly sparks joy in your life.

It is now time to hit the refresh button on your life. It's the perfect time to pause, reflect on your journey, and decide what truly matters to you. What are your priorities?

It's important to spend time with people who are not from work, have hobbies and interests outside of your job, and nurture your unique qualities beyond your professional life.

It can be a bit puzzling at times. Without the usual routine or children causing chaos, one might ask, "What should I do next?"

This opportunity is your key to exploring, experimenting, and discovering new passions. Here are some tips to help you progress smoothly:

- **Take a life inventory:** Ask yourself this question. What would you do if money and fear weren't an issue? Dream big!

- **Stay connected:** Don't let loneliness crash the retirement party. Reach out to your friends, join clubs, volunteer, or mingle with new faces. Your social circle will help you fight against boredom!

- **Get real with yourself:** It's time to unleash your authentic self. Try new things, meet new people, and seek out new adventures. The real treasure lies within, so go on and discover who the new you is!

- **Keep on learning:** Retirement isn't a ticket to stagnation. Embrace learning like it's the fountain of youth! Whether it's picking up a new skill or mastering a hobby, keep that brain buzzing with excitement.

The Stability Phase

Reaching the stability phase is like finding that perfect spot on a hammock where you can just relax and sway without a care in the world. After all the emotional upheaval of retirement, you're finally settling into your groove.

In this phase, you're not just coasting; you're thriving. You've embraced your retirement identity like a badge of honor and crafted a daily routine that's as cozy as your favorite sweater. Maybe you're diving into hobbies you never had time for before or reconnecting with loved ones who bring laughter to your life. It's all about finding that sweet spot where every day feels like a gift.

But what's next? How do you keep this momentum going? Here are some tips to keep you soaring through this phase like an expert:

- **Protect your retirement purpose:** You've put in the work to discover what truly sets your soul on fire in retirement. Now, it's time to nurture that flame. Keep those meaningful activities front and center, and take small steps every day that align with your newfound purpose.

- **Prioritize self-care:** You are the leader of your retirement journey, so it is important to prioritize your well-being. Dedicate time to care for yourself, focusing on both your mental and physical health. Whether it involves a daily walk, a yoga practice, or simply enjoying a peaceful moment with a good book, ensure that self-care remains a top priority.

- **Embrace challenges:** Life's adventures don't stop just because you've retired. Keep pushing yourself outside of your comfort zone and be open to whatever comes your way. Trust in your ability to handle whatever life throws at you, and remember, every challenge is just another opportunity for growth.

- **Focus on growth:** Retirement isn't the end of the road; it's just a new one. Keep that growth mindset alive and kicking by continuously seeking opportunities to learn and evolve, like picking up a new skill or tackling a passion project. Never stop reaching for the stars.

- **Be fully present:** In a world that's constantly buzzing with distractions, it's easy to lose sight of the beauty in the little moments. Take time each day to ground yourself in the present, whether it's through meditation, exercise, or simply savoring your morning coffee. Trust me, life is so much sweeter when you're fully present for it.

The Legacy Phase

This marks the beginning of an exciting journey. With decades of valuable experience, it is now your moment to impart your wisdom to the world. Let's talk about how you can make this phase the most fulfilling and impactful one yet:

- **Beyond material wealth:** Legacy in retirement isn't just about money or possessions; it's about leaving a lasting impact on the world that goes beyond material wealth. It's about the values you instill in others, the memories you create, and the positive influence you have on people's lives. It's the imprint you leave on future generations and the mark you make on society through your actions and contributions. Legacy in retirement is about shaping a better world for those who come after you and being remembered for the positive difference you made during your lifetime.

- **Giving back to your community:** Engaging in volunteer work isn't just about staying active and involved; it's like a social superglue that bonds you to your community. Whether you're helping out at a soup kitchen, tutoring students, or cuddling furry friends at an animal shelter, the chances to make a difference are endless. These activities let you give back to society, grow personally, and find fulfillment along the way.

- **Passing on wisdom through mentoring:** With decades of experience under your belt, mentoring is like a perfectly tailored suit that never goes out of style. Whether you're doling out career wisdom to fresh-faced professionals or passing on life hacks to your grandkids, mentoring lets you sprinkle a little stardust of knowledge and make a lasting impact on someone else's journey.

- **Living your values every day:** Legacy isn't just about the grand gestures; it's about the tiny ripples of kindness, the sprinkle of compassion, and the dash of generosity you add to life's recipe. By seasoning your everyday interactions with these flavors, you're not just leaving a mark on the world; you're creating a legacy worth savoring for generations to come.

- **Finding fulfillment in passion pursuits:** Cultivating a sense of purpose in retirement involves staying true to yourself and following your passions. Whether it's painting vibrant landscapes, tending to a flourishing garden, penning captivating stories, or embarking on exciting adventures around the world, find what brings you joy and pursue it with gusto.

- **Embrace new adventures and reinvention:** Retirement isn't the end; it's a new beginning full of exciting possibilities waiting to be explored. Embrace new experiences, seek uncharted hobbies, and fearlessly reinvent yourself. Remember, it's never too late to uncover the treasures that life has in store for you.

- **Making the most of precious time:** The legacy phase of retirement is like being handed the baton in a relay race—it's your time to sprint toward the finish line of life with style and flair. Remember, life's a grand adventure, so grab your popcorn, sit back, and enjoy the show. You're the star of your own legacy production!

In the end, the legacy phase of retirement is all about making the most of this precious time we have left. So go out there, embrace life with open arms, and leave behind a legacy that you can be proud of. After all, you've earned it!

As we conclude this chapter, allow me to emphasize: Retirement entails more than simply completing phases; it involves embracing each stage, gaining insights from them, and preparing for the upcoming chapter.

So, what comes next? You are on the verge of exploring the incredible realm of nurturing a positive mindset! You are preparing to equip yourself with the most potent asset in your retirement arsenal: your mindset.

Get ready to change your perspective on negative thoughts, welcome the strength of positivity, and learn how developing the right mindset can transform even the gloomiest retirement day into an exciting adventure. We will explore effective strategies that will leave you motivated, empowered, and prepared to face whatever challenges retirement may bring your way.

CHAPTER 3:
CULTIVATING A POSITIVE MINDSET

As someone preparing to retire or a seasoned retiree, this phase of life is filled with endless possibilities, discoveries, and adventures. Retirement is your chance to redefine yourself, explore your passions, and embrace the joy of living on your terms.

However, transitioning into retirement isn't just about financial planning and leisurely activities; it's also about nurturing a positive mindset that will empower you to thrive in this new chapter. Retirees today are not simply fading into the background; instead, they're seizing the opportunity to live their best lives yet.

In this chapter, we will explore practical strategies and techniques designed to assist you in sustaining a positive outlook and overcoming any mental obstacles that may surface on your journey. While retirement may present challenges, by adopting the appropriate mindset, you can confront them with elegance and resilience.

Practicing Gratitude and Reframing Negative Thoughts

We have discussed some of the challenges that retirement can bring. One of the most powerful tools you have at your disposal to navigate these is the practice of gratitude and the ability to reframe negative thoughts.

Gratitude isn't just a fleeting feeling of appreciation; it's a mindset, a way of seeing the world through a lens of abundance rather than scarcity. As a retiree, you have a wealth of experiences to draw upon, and by embracing gratitude, you can unlock the full potential of this chapter in your life.

Why is gratitude so important in retirement, you may ask? Well, let me share a few compelling reasons with you:

- **Fostering positivity:**

  o **Shift in focus:** Gratitude serves as a powerful lens through which to view the world. By consciously acknowledging and appreciating the blessings in your life, no matter how small, you redirect your attention from negativity to positivity.

  o **Mood enhancement:** Embracing a mindset of gratitude uplifts your mood and brightens your outlook on life. Instead of dwelling on challenges or shortcomings, you cultivate an attitude of appreciation that fosters joy and contentment.

  o **Psychological well-being:** Studies have shown that practicing gratitude is linked to improved mental health outcomes, including reduced stress, anxiety, and depression (Reid, 2024). By nurturing a sense of gratitude, you enhance your overall psychological well-being in retirement.

- **Cultivating resilience:**

  o **Facing adversity:** Retirement brings its own set of challenges, from health issues to financial concerns and beyond. Cultivating gratitude equips you with the resilience to navigate these obstacles with grace and tenacity.

  o **Finding silver linings:** Through the practice of gratitude, you train your mind to identify silver linings even in the midst of adversity. Rather than succumbing to despair, you develop the ability to extract valuable lessons and growth opportunities from life's challenges.

  o **Strength and empowerment:** Gratitude empowers you to bounce back stronger than ever before. By acknowledging your blessings and strengths, you cultivate inner resilience that enables you to weather life's storms with grace and fortitude.

- **Enhancing relationships:**

  o **Deepening connections:** Gratitude is a powerful catalyst for strengthening relationships in retirement. When you express appreciation and gratitude toward your loved ones, you deepen your connections and foster a sense of mutual respect and admiration.

o **Positive feedback loop:** Acts of gratitude create a positive feedback loop within relationships. Expressing gratitude cultivates feelings of warmth and reciprocity, prompting others to respond in kind. This cycle of appreciation enriches and sustains meaningful relationships.

o **Building trust and intimacy:** Openly expressing gratitude fosters trust and intimacy within relationships. It creates a safe and nurturing environment where individuals feel valued, respected, and understood, enhancing the quality of interpersonal connections in retirement.

In essence, gratitude serves as a cornerstone of well-being in retirement, enriching your life in myriad ways. When you foster positivity, cultivate resilience, and enhance relationships through the practice of gratitude, you unlock the full potential of this transformative mindset. Embrace gratitude as a guiding principle in your retirement journey, and watch as it infuses every aspect of your life with meaning, fulfillment, and joy.

Now, let's talk about reframing negative thoughts. Negative thoughts are like weeds in the garden of your mind—if left unchecked, they can choke out the beautiful flowers of positivity and growth. You have the power to uproot these weeds and plant seeds of positivity in their place.

Reframing negative thoughts is all about challenging the stories we tell ourselves and finding alternative, more empowering perspectives. For example, instead of viewing retirement as a time of loss—loss of identity, loss of purpose, loss of routine—reframe it as a time of liberation, a blank canvas upon which you can paint the masterpiece of your dreams.

Here are a few strategies to help you reframe negative thoughts:

• **Practice self-compassion:** Be gentle with yourself. Acknowledge that negative thoughts are a natural part of being human, but don't let them define you. Treat yourself with the same warmth and understanding that you would offer to a good friend or someone you loved facing similar challenges.

- **Challenge negative assumptions**: When you catch yourself falling into a spiral of negativity, pause and ask yourself: *Is this thought really true? What evidence do I have to support it?* Often, you'll find that your negative assumptions are based on faulty logic or outdated beliefs.

- **Focus on solutions**: Instead of dwelling on problems, shift your focus to solutions. Ask yourself: "*What can I do to overcome this challenge? What resources or support do I have at my disposal?*" By taking proactive steps toward finding solutions, you reclaim your agency and empower yourself to create positive change.

Tips on Incorporating Gratitude Practices Into Daily Life

Practicing gratitude and reframing negative thoughts are essential habits for any happy retiree. They have the power to transform your retirement from mere existence to true fulfillment and joy. Here are some tips to help you incorporate gratitude practices into your daily life:

- **Start a gratitude journal:** Take a few minutes each day to jot down three things you're grateful for. They can be big or small, profound or seemingly trivial. The act of writing them down helps solidify the feeling of gratitude in your mind and heart.

- **Morning gratitude ritual:** Begin each day by setting an intention to notice and appreciate the blessings in your life. Whether it's the warmth of the sun on your face, the aroma of freshly brewed coffee, or the sound of birds outside your window, consciously acknowledge the beauty around you.

- **Express appreciation to others and yourself:** Make it a habit to express gratitude to the people in your life. A heartfelt "thank you" to your spouse for their love and support, a note of appreciation to a friend for their kindness, or a word of thanks to the cashier at the grocery store can brighten someone's day and deepen your own sense of connection. It is important to allow yourself the same appreciation. Be mindful of your amazing qualities and what positive attributes you bring to the table.

- **Practice mindfulness:** Cultivate mindfulness by paying attention to the present moment with openness and curiosity. Notice the sensations in your body, the thoughts passing through your mind, and the emotions that arise. When you encounter challenges or difficulties, approach them with a spirit of curiosity and compassion rather than judgment.

- **Shift your perspective:** Instead of dwelling on what's lacking or going wrong, focus on what you've learned, how you've grown, or the silver linings. Every setback is an opportunity for growth and resilience.

I encourage you to embrace these habits wholeheartedly and watch as they enrich every aspect of your life in retirement.

Developing Resilience and Adapting to Life Changes

Let's talk about resilience. It's the secret that can make your retirement not just enjoyable but deeply satisfying. Resilience isn't about being unaffected by challenges; it's about bouncing back stronger and wiser when life throws curveballs your way.

Resilience means being able to handle tough situations well. It's about bouncing back from setbacks, staying calm during hard times, and becoming stronger through challenges. Resilience involves mental, emotional, and social skills that help people deal with problems in a positive way. It's not about avoiding problems but about building inner strength to face and conquer them effectively.

During retirement, you're transitioning from a structured work life to a more flexible, open-ended existence. This shift can be both exhilarating and daunting. So, how can you become resilient?:

- **Mindset mastery:** Start cultivating that positive mindset. Embrace the belief that challenges are opportunities for growth.

No more viewing retirement as an end; see it as a new beginning filled with incredible possibilities.

- **Stay connected:** Social connections are necessary for resilience. Nurture relationships with friends, family, and your community. Join clubs, volunteer, or pursue hobbies that bring you into contact with like-minded people. These connections will provide support and perspective during times of change.

- **Flexibility and adaptability:** Embrace flexibility in your plans and expectations. Life rarely goes according to script, and that's okay! Stay open to detours and unexpected opportunities that come your way. Being flexible allows you to adapt to changing circumstances with ease.

- **Self-care:** Take care of your physical, emotional, and mental well-being. Prioritize activities that rejuvenate and replenish your energy. Whether it's exercise, meditation, or simply indulging in your favorite pastimes, make self-care a non-negotiable part of your routine.

- **Continuous learning:** Keep your mind sharp by pursuing new interests and learning experiences. Attend workshops or enroll in courses that stimulate your intellect. Lifelong learning not only keeps you engaged but also enhances your adaptability to new situations.

Now, let's talk about the benefits of embracing flexibility and seizing new opportunities in retirement.

Flexibility allows you to approach life with a sense of freedom and adventure. Instead of feeling constrained by rigid schedules and expectations, you have the liberty to explore your passions, travel to new places, and pursue exciting activities. Embracing flexibility opens doors to a world of possibilities, ensuring that each day is filled with excitement and fulfillment.

Moreover, seizing new opportunities keeps your mind active and your spirit youthful. It's never too late to reinvent yourself and discover untapped potential within.

Finding Purpose and Setting Meaningful Goals in Retirement

Today's retirees are vibrant, active individuals ready to make the most of this precious time. And it all starts with finding your purpose.

You might be asking yourself: *How can I find my purpose in retirement?*:

- **Reflect on your passions:** Dedicate some time to consider what genuinely fills your heart and makes you content. Do you like volunteering and giving back to a cause that means a lot to you? Can you remember a passion you had when you were younger that has been put on the back burner? Perhaps you were passionate about an instrument you played in high school or loved to cook and have thought about taking some classes.

- **Discover new hobbies:** Retirement is the perfect time to explore new avenues. When we are busy working, we tend to put off those things that are, well, fun! Instead of saving travel for those once-a-year summer vacations, why not explore places in your own country you've always wanted to see? Whether you have an interest in learning a new language, taking a class in photography, or pushing outside your comfort zone to try a strength training class, retirement offers the opportunity to expand your hobbies and meet new people!

- **Give back:** Volunteering can be incredibly rewarding and is a fantastic way to find purpose in retirement. There are many ways to kick off that volunteering journey. If you love animals, check in with your local animal shelter. If you coach your own children in youth sports, visit local youth teams and inquire about non-parent coaching opportunities. If you're passionate about the environment, visit your local city website and ask about tree planting days or park garbage cleanup.

So, how exactly do we set meaningful goals?:

- **Align with your values:** When setting goals in retirement, it's essential to align them with your personal values. Ask yourself what truly matters to you, and let those values guide your decisions. Whether it's spending more time with family, prioritizing health and wellness, or pursuing lifelong dreams, ensure that your goals resonate with your core beliefs.

- **Start small:** Setting achievable goals is key to staying motivated and maintaining momentum. It is easy to get overwhelmed if you set a goal that is too large. For example, you may be motivated to live a healthier lifestyle. To kick it off, maybe you set a goal of climbing a large mountain peak in your area. If walking is not your favorite activity, you may want to break this down into smaller steps so you are not setting yourself up for failure. Break larger goals down into smaller, actionable steps, and celebrate each milestone along the way. Whether it's learning a new skill, decluttering your home, or planning a dream vacation, taking small, consistent actions will keep you moving forward.

- **Create a vision board:** Visualizing your goals can be incredibly powerful. Consider creating a vision board filled with images and words that represent your aspirations. Place it somewhere prominent where you'll see it every day, serving as a constant reminder of what you're working toward.

Remember, retirement is a time to start new beginnings and pursue your passions with vigor. By finding purpose and setting meaningful goals aligned with your values and interests, you'll unlock a world of possibilities and create a retirement filled with joy, fulfillment, and purpose.

Building Self-Confidence and Embracing Personal Growth

Retirement is a golden opportunity for reinvention, self-discovery, and continuous growth. As retirees today, you redefine what it means to age gracefully, and that includes nurturing your self-confidence and embracing personal development at every turn.

Let's look closer at how you can build self-confidence:

- **Embrace your uniqueness:** Understand that you bring a wealth of experiences, skills, and wisdom to the table. Embrace your individuality and recognize your value in every situation.

- **Challenge negative self-talk:** We all have that inner critic, but it's time to challenge its authority. Replace negative self-talk with affirmations of your worth and capabilities. Remind yourself of past successes and strengths.

- **Set realistic goals:** Remember, you can avoid failure by breaking down big aspirations into smaller, achievable goals. With each accomplishment, your confidence will grow, propelling you forward to tackle even more significant challenges.

- **Step out of your comfort zone:** Growth happens when we push ourselves beyond what feels comfortable. Take calculated risks, try new activities, and explore unfamiliar territories. Each step outside your comfort zone is a victory for your confidence.

- **Celebrate your wins:** Don't downplay your achievements, no matter how small they may seem. Celebrate every milestone reached and use these victories as fuel to push you toward even greater accomplishments.

Here are time strategies to embrace personal growth opportunities:

- **Continue to learn:** Retirement is the perfect time to indulge your curiosity and pursue new interests. Enroll in classes, join discussion groups, or simply check out books or podcasts on topics that intrigue you.

- **Become resilient:** As discussed, challenges are inevitable, but how we respond to them shapes our growth. Remember to cultivate resilience by viewing setbacks as opportunities for learning and self-improvement. Adaptability is a hallmark of personal development.

- **Seek feedback and support:** Surround yourself with those who uplift and inspire you. Seek feedback from trusted friends, mentors, or even professional coaches who can provide guidance and encouragement on your journey of personal growth.

- **Practice mindfulness:** Take time to reflect on your experiences, emotions, and aspirations. Mindfulness cultivates self-awareness and opens the door to deeper self-discovery. Through mindfulness practices such as meditation or journaling, you can navigate your inner landscape with clarity and purpose.

- **Stay open to change**: Embrace the beauty of life's ever-changing nature. Be open to new possibilities, opportunities, and perspectives. The willingness to adapt and evolve ensures that you continue growing and thriving throughout your retirement years.

Managing Expectations and Embracing Flexibility

So, why is managing expectations and embracing flexibility so important in retirement?

First, it's about maintaining a positive outlook. When we hold onto rigid expectations, we set ourselves up for disappointment if things don't go exactly as planned. By cultivating a mindset of flexibility, we're better equipped to roll with the punches and find joy in the unexpected.

Moreover, flexibility fosters resilience. Retirement, like any other phase of life, comes with its own set of challenges. Whether it's adjusting to a fixed income, dealing with health issues, or navigating changes in relationships, flexibility allows us to adapt and thrive in the face of adversity.

Here are some things to consider (Senior Experts, 2022):

- Developing a realistic view of retirement is important. Retirement isn't always carefree and relaxing.

- Most retirees state that the primary challenge in retirement is the absence of a clear sense of purpose.

- Studies show that the retirees who have planned for and anticipated the retirement adjustment process are the most successful.

- The retirees who were most successful adjusted their expectations, found new sources of meaning and purpose, and stayed active in their lives.

Balancing Expectations and Reality in Retirement

One of the challenges of transitioning into retirement is recognizing the delicate equilibrium between your expectations and the actuality. Retirees can take steps to facilitate their adjustment to retirement, including:

- **Cultivate social connections:** Prioritize building and maintaining relationships with friends, family, and community members. When you nurture social connections, you can create a supportive network that enhances your overall well-being and enriches your retirement experience.

- **Seize opportunities:** Take advantage of the chances around you, such as volunteering. We have discussed how contributing your time and skills not only benefits the community but also provides a sense of purpose and satisfaction in your retirement years.

Finding a new purpose in life during retirement is a significant benefit and a goal worth pursuing!

As you get closer to retiring, you might imagine how you want your life to be during this new phase. While it may seem perfect in your thoughts, the actual experience can be quite different.

If you dream of relaxing on a beach in paradise, reading a good book, and living a carefree life during retirement, it's time to start working toward that goal. If your perfect idea of retirement is traveling the world or spending more time with family, plan for that.

Remember, retirement is not the end of the road; it's a new beginning filled with infinite possibilities. By managing expectations and embracing flexibility, you'll not only navigate this exciting chapter with ease but also discover a newfound sense of joy, fulfillment, and purpose along the way.

As you reflect on the insights and strategies shared in this chapter, I encourage you to carry them forward into your daily life. Embrace each day with gratitude, seek out the silver linings, and approach challenges with resilience and optimism. By doing so, you'll unlock the true potential of your retirement years and discover newfound joy in every moment.

Now, as we turn the page to our next chapter, get ready to start this exciting time of exploration and discovery. In the upcoming chapter, we'll dig deep into the art of finding new interests and hobbies, igniting your passion, and uncovering hidden talents you never knew you had.

CHAPTER 4:
FINDING NEW INTERESTS AND HOBBIES

Finding new interests and hobbies isn't merely a pastime; it's a pathway to personal fulfillment and growth. It's about discovering facets of yourself you never knew existed and nurturing your well-being in the process. From cultivating a green thumb in your garden to unleashing your inner artist through painting or pottery, the avenues for exploration are as vast as your imagination.

Throughout this chapter, we'll learn practical strategies and time-tested advice to help you navigate this exciting terrain. We'll explore the importance of identifying your unique interests and passions, providing a compass to guide you toward activities that resonate with your soul.

But it's not just about solitary pursuits; it's about building connections and fostering a sense of community. The bonds formed through shared interests can enrich your life in ways you never thought possible.

As we journey together through this chapter, remember that finding new interests and hobbies is not just an item on your retirement to-do list; it's a mindset, a commitment to living life to the fullest.

Identifying Personal Interests and Passions

Retirement is an opportunity to rediscover yourself, to reignite the flames of curiosity and passion that the demands of work and daily life may have dimmed.

Let's start with a simple question: What really excites you? What gets you out of bed in the morning and makes you happy?

Self-reflection is similar to shining a light into your inner self. It involves pausing, blocking those outside distractions, and tuning in to your inner thoughts. Retirement provides the perfect chance to explore this introspective process deeply without the distractions of work.

So, how do we begin? Start by carving out some quiet time for yourself. This could be a few minutes each day or a longer period dedicated to reflection and contemplation. Find a peaceful space where you feel comfortable and free from distractions. Grab a journal or a notebook, and let's embark on this journey together.

Begin by asking yourself some fundamental questions:

- What activities bring me the greatest sense of joy and fulfillment?

- What hobbies or interests have I always wanted to pursue but never had the time for?

- What experiences have left a lasting impression on me?

- When do I feel most alive and engaged?

As you ponder these questions, pay attention to the thoughts and feelings that arise within you. Notice any patterns or recurring themes. Perhaps you'll uncover a long-forgotten passion for culinary exploration, community activism, or adventure sports. Maybe you'll realize that spending time with family brings you the greatest joy. Whatever it may be, embrace it wholeheartedly.

Remember, retirement is your time to explore, experiment, and indulge in the things that bring you genuine happiness. This is the time to try new and exciting things. This is your chance to write the next chapter of your life exactly as you envision it.

Once you've identified your personal interests and passions, the next step is to cultivate them intentionally. Schedule regular time in your calendar to pursue these activities. Seek out workshops, classes, or events where you can learn and grow.

Above all, approach this journey with an open heart and a curious mind. Welcome the process of self-discovery with enthusiasm and optimism. Your retirement years are a precious gift, and it's up to you to make the most of them.

In the words of Henry David Thoreau, "Go confidently in the direction of your dreams. Live the life you have imagined."

Trying New Experiences

Stepping out of your comfort zone is like opening a door to a world of endless opportunities. It's about pushing your boundaries, challenging yourself, and embracing growth. In retirement, this becomes even more crucial as it keeps your mind sharp, your spirit young, and your heart full.

By welcoming new challenges, you're not just trying something different; you're rewiring your brain, fostering resilience, and boosting your confidence. Whether it's learning a new language, mastering a musical instrument, or taking up cooking classes you've always been curious about, each new experience expands your horizons and adds color to your life.

Suggestions for Trying a Variety of Hobbies and Experiences

The key to unlocking a world of possibilities in retirement is to cast a wide net and try a variety of hobbies and experiences.

Here are a few suggestions to get you started:

- **Creative pursuits**: Channel your artistic talents into creative outlets such as filmmaking, graphic design, or music production. Take classes, workshops, or online courses to hone your skills and express yourself through various mediums.

- **Entrepreneurship**: Consider starting a small business or pursuing a passion project you've always dreamed of. Whether it's launching a boutique bakery, creating an online shop for handmade crafts, or offering consulting services in your area of expertise, entrepreneurship can bring fulfillment and financial rewards.

- **Fitness challenges**: Set ambitious fitness goals and challenge yourself to new heights. Sign up for marathons, triathlons, or obstacle course races to push your limits and stay in peak physical condition.

- **Travel**: Embark on adventures near and far, whether it's exploring exotic destinations, embarking on a road trip, or simply discovering hidden gems in your own backyard. Travel opens your eyes to different cultures, cuisines, and perspectives, enriching your life in ways you never imagined.

- **Volunteer work and community engagement:** By immersing yourself in activities that serve others, you not only contribute positively to society but also open yourself up to new opportunities and interests. These interactions can spark curiosity and lead you to discover new hobbies and passions.

- **Sustainable living**: Embrace a lifestyle focused on sustainability and environmental stewardship. Start a garden, learn to compost, or participate in conservation projects in your community. Adopting eco-friendly habits not only benefits the planet but also promotes personal well-being.

- **Tech innovation**: Stay at the forefront of technology by exploring emerging trends and innovations. Experiment with virtual reality, drone photography, or 3D printing to discover new ways of engaging with the world and expressing your creativity.

- **Spiritual exploration**: Start down a path of self-discovery and spiritual growth through practices such as meditation, yoga, or mindfulness. Attend retreats, workshops, or spiritual gatherings to deepen your understanding of yourself and the universe.

Overcoming Fears and Reservations

It's natural to feel apprehensive about trying new activities, especially as you get older. It's important to understand that growth often occurs just outside of our comfort zone. Here are some tips for overcoming fears and reservations:

- **Identifying fears:** First, you should take a moment to recognize and accept your fears without judgment. It's okay to feel nervous about trying something new— you're stepping out of your comfort zone, and that takes courage. Start by asking yourself: *What am I afraid of? Is it failure? Rejection? Embarrassment? Loss of control?* Understanding the root of your fear can help you address it head-on. Take a closer look at them. Are they based on facts or assumptions? Often, our fears are inflated by our imagination. By examining them closely, you might realize they're not as daunting as they seem.

- **Focus on the excitement:** Instead of dwelling on what could go wrong, focus on the excitement and possibilities that await. Visualize yourself succeeding and enjoying the journey. Challenge those negative thoughts by looking at the positive rather than the negative.

- **Start small:** Break down daunting tasks into smaller, manageable steps. Gradually ease into new experiences, allowing yourself to build confidence along the way.

- **Embrace the learning process:** Remember that every beginner was once a novice. Embrace the learning process with humility and curiosity, knowing that mistakes and setbacks are natural parts of the journey.

- **Seek support:** Don't be afraid to lean on friends, family, or fellow enthusiasts for support and encouragement. Surround yourself with positive influences who believe in your ability to thrive.

Joining Clubs and Social Groups

The CDC reports that 1 in every 4 individuals aged 65 and over suffer from social isolation. They also claim social isolation may lead to significant health issues, including (*Loneliness and Social Isolation*, 2021):

- high blood pressure

- heart disease

- obesity

- weakened immune system

- anxiety

- depression

- cognitive deterioration

- Alzheimer's disease

Alternatively, when retirees participate in meaningful activities that promote connection, these risks are significantly reduced. Studies have found better cognitive function, enhanced mood, and longer lifespans for retirees who take part in social and group activities (Statistics Canada, 2015).

Let's explore even more advantages of joining these communities and how they can enrich your retirement experience:

- **Fostering connections and building community:** One of the greatest benefits of joining clubs and social groups is the opportunity to connect with like-minded people who share your interests and passions. These connections not only provide companionship but also create a sense of belonging and camaraderie, which are essential for a fulfilling retirement.

- **Recommendations for local services:** Whether you're in need of a reliable plumber, a trustworthy mechanic, or a reputable healthcare provider, your fellow club members can be an excellent source of recommendations. As active members of the community, they've likely utilized various services and can provide firsthand insights and advice to help you make informed decisions.

- **Advice on navigating retirement-related challenges:** Retirement may bring about its fair share of challenges, from adjusting to a new routine to managing financial concerns. Being part of a support group allows you to tap into the collective wisdom and experiences of others who have walked a similar path. Maybe you're grappling with healthcare decisions, estate planning, or finding meaningful ways to fill your time. Here, you'll find compassionate ears and valuable advice within your community.

- **Access to helpful tools and resources:** Many clubs and support groups offer access to workshops, seminars, and informational materials designed specifically for retirees. From financial planning seminars to health and wellness workshops, these resources provide practical guidance and tools to help you thrive in retirement. Additionally, some groups may have partnerships with local organizations or businesses, offering exclusive discounts or services to members.

- **Enhancing the retirement experience:** Participating in clubs and social groups can add a whole new dimension to your retirement experience. Not only do they provide opportunities for social interaction and intellectual stimulation, but they also offer a platform for learning and growth. Whether you're picking up a new hobby, expanding your knowledge, or simply enjoying the company of others, these shared experiences can bring immense joy and fulfillment to your life.

Now, you might be wondering how to get started on this journey. Here are a few tips to help you along the way:

- Revisit your list of your interests and hobbies. Remind yourself of the activities that bring you joy and fulfillment.

- Reach out to local community centers, libraries, or online forums to discover clubs and groups in your area.

- Attend introductory meetings or events to get a sense of the group dynamics and see if it's a good fit for you.

By actively engaging in these communities, you'll not only enhance your social life but also create lasting friendships and memories that will enrich your life for years to come.

Finding Creative Outlets and Engaging in Artistic Pursuits

Retirees today are vibrant, active, and full of zest for life. And what better way to channel that energy than through creative expression?

Engaging in creative outlets and artistic pursuits during retirement offers a multitude of benefits beyond mere entertainment. It's a powerful means of self-expression, allowing you to communicate thoughts, feelings, and experiences in unique and meaningful ways. Whether it's painting, writing, pottery, photography, or music, there's an artistic medium out there waiting for you to explore.

But why should you bother with creativity in retirement? Let me tell you—it's not just about filling idle hours. Creative activities have the remarkable ability to stimulate your mind, foster personal growth, and enhance overall well-being.

First, creativity keeps your brain sharp. Just like physical exercise is essential for maintaining a healthy body, engaging in creative endeavors exercises your brain, keeping it agile and adaptable. It challenges you to think outside the box, solve problems creatively, and embrace new perspectives—all invaluable skills for moving through life in retirement.

Moreover, artistic pursuits offer a sense of purpose and fulfillment. They provide an outlet for self-discovery and exploration, allowing you to uncover hidden talents and passions you may not have known existed. Whether you're experienced or new to art, creating can bring joy from start to finish.

Now, you might be wondering, "But where do I start?" There's a world of creative activities waiting for you to experience.

Here are some ideas to ignite your creativity:

- **Try Something New:**
    - **Experiment with mediums:** Explore various artistic mediums and techniques. Attend a pottery class to mold

clay into beautiful creations, or try your hand at sculpture. Embrace the thrill of discovery as you venture into uncharted territory, discovering hidden talents you never knew you had.

- **Attend workshops:** Join workshops or classes focused on creative endeavors. Whether it's painting, writing, or even learning an instrument, these structured settings provide guidance and support as you dive into new realms of creativity.

- **Step out of your comfort zone:** Challenge yourself to try activities you've never considered before. From salsa dancing to aerial yoga, embrace the opportunity to push your boundaries and uncover new passions.

- **Capture Moments:**
  - **Photography adventures:** Grab your camera or smartphone and embark on photography expeditions. Explore the beauty of nature, the intricacies of urban landscapes, or the candid moments of everyday life. Photography not only preserves memories but also encourages you to see the world through a new lens, appreciating the beauty in the ordinary.

  - **Create visual journals:** Document your retirement adventures through visual journals or scrapbooks. Combine photographs with handwritten notes, ticket stubs, and mementos to create personalized keepsakes that tell the story of your journey.

- **Embrace DIY Projects:**
  - **Get crafty:** Enter the world of do-it-yourself (DIY) crafts and projects. Whether it's woodworking, gardening, knitting, or jewelry making, embrace the satisfaction of creating something with your own hands. Not only do DIY projects provide a creative outlet, but they also offer a sense of accomplishment and pride as you see your ideas come to fruition.

- o **Join crafting communities:** Connect with fellow DIY enthusiasts by joining crafting communities or online forums. Share ideas, tips, and inspiration with like-minded individuals who share your passion for creativity and craftsmanship.

- **Write Your Story:**

  - o **Start a journal:** Begin each day by jotting down your thoughts, reflections, and experiences in a journal. Use writing as a tool for self-discovery and expression, capturing the essence of your retirement journey.

  - o **Explore creative writing:** Experiment with various forms of creative writing, from short stories and poetry to essays and memoirs. Your life experiences are rich with stories waiting to be told, and retirement offers the perfect opportunity to unleash your storytelling prowess.

  - o **Share your wisdom:** Consider sharing your writing with others through blogging, community publications, or even self-publishing. Your unique perspective and insights can inspire and resonate with readers, leaving a lasting impact beyond your own retirement years.

Remember, the key to embracing new experiences in retirement is to approach them with an open mind and a sense of curiosity. Whether you're painting a masterpiece, capturing moments through photography, crafting handmade treasures, or writing your life story, each creative endeavor enriches your retirement journey and leaves a legacy of inspiration for years to come. So, don't hesitate—jump in and let your creativity soar!

Finally, let's not overlook the therapeutic benefits of artistic pursuits. Creating art can be incredibly cathartic, offering a release valve for stress and anxiety. It allows you to express emotions that may be difficult to articulate verbally, providing a sense of relief and emotional well-being.

In retirement, embracing creativity means embracing life fully. It involves finding joy in creating, excitement in discovering, and satisfaction in expressing yourself genuinely. So go ahead, pick up that paintbrush, strum that guitar, or write that poem. Your retirement journey is yours to shape—and creativity is your passport to limitless possibilities.

Leisure Activities and Personal Growth

Retirement offers the luxury of time, but managing it effectively is key. Balancing leisure activities with personal growth ensures you enjoy your newfound freedom while also nurturing your mind, body, and spirit. Think of it as tending to your holistic well-being.

Leisure isn't just about doing nothing; it's about relaxing and refueling. Spending time with loved ones, doing hobbies, or traveling can recharge you and make you happy. Enjoy these activities without feeling guilty.

Strategies for Effective Time Management

Time management is crucial for harmonizing leisure and personal growth pursuits. Start by creating a weekly schedule that allocates dedicated time for both. Treat these commitments with the same importance as you would a doctor's appointment or a social outing.

Consider batching similar activities together to maximize efficiency. For example, designate mornings for personal growth endeavors like reading or learning a new language and reserve afternoons for leisurely pursuits such as gardening or painting.

Be flexible and open to adjusting your schedule as needed. Retirement is about freedom, after all. Allow yourself to indulge in spontaneous adventures or pursue unexpected opportunities that arise.

The Benefits of Personal Growth in Retirement

Personal growth isn't just a buzzword—it's the secret sauce to a fulfilling retirement. Continuously challenging yourself intellectually, emotionally, and spiritually keeps your mind sharp and your spirit vibrant.

Personal development also nurtures a feeling of purpose. As you start new adventures and expand your horizons, you'll discover talents and passions. Your contributions to society can take on new meaning in retirement.

As you've learned, discovering new hobbies can enrich your life in countless ways. Embrace this opportunity to explore your interests, ignite your creativity, and connect with like-minded individuals who share your passions.

But our journey doesn't end here. In the next chapter, we'll discuss the importance of prioritizing physical health during retirement. Your health is key, and by making conscious choices to stay active and fit, you'll not only enhance your quality of life but also ensure that you're able to fully enjoy all the experiences that retirement has to offer.

So get ready to start the next leg of our adventure together. Get excited about prioritizing your physical well-being and unlocking even more vitality and energy to fuel your retirement dreams.

CHAPTER 5:
PRIORITIZING YOUR PHYSICAL HEALTH

On to a chapter that celebrates the vessel that carries you through each and every day: your body. In retirement, it's more crucial than ever to tend to this remarkable instrument with care and intention. As you start on this new phase of life, let's explore the essential practices that will ensure your physical well-being remains strong, vibrant, and ready for all the adventures that lie ahead.

Your body deserves your attention, respect, and nurturing. Within these pages, we'll explore how to maintain physical health: exercise, nutrition, and preventive healthcare practices.

Exercise isn't just about fitting into a certain size of jeans or impressing others with your athleticism. It's about honoring your body's need for movement, strength, and vitality. I'll guide you through designing an exercise routine that suits your unique needs and abilities, ensuring that staying active becomes a joyful part of your daily routine.

Nutrition is the fuel that powers your body and mind, influencing everything from your energy levels to your mood. I'll delve into the role of nutrition in promoting overall well-being, offering practical tips and delicious recipes to nourish your body.

Preventive healthcare practices are the cornerstone of longevity and vitality. By taking proactive measures to safeguard your health, you can prevent common ailments and enjoy a life of wellness. I'll equip you with the knowledge and tools to prioritize preventive care and make informed decisions about your health.

As we age, our bodies inevitably undergo changes, and it's important to adapt gracefully to these shifts. We'll explore how to move through physical changes and limitations in retirement with resilience, positivity, and a spirit of self-compassion.

By prioritizing your physical health, you're not just adding years to your life; you're adding life to your years.

Designing an Exercise Routine Suitable for Retirees

Regular exercise brings many incredible benefits to your retirement years. First, exercise is exactly what your cardiovascular health needs. It keeps your heart strong and pumping efficiently, reducing the risk of heart disease and stroke. Exercise remains the best way to improve arterial function with aging (Murray et al., 2023). Isn't that amazing? By simply moving your body, you're safeguarding your most vital organ.

Regular exercise also boosts your strength and flexibility. This means you'll find it easier to perform everyday tasks, whether it's carrying groceries, playing with your grandchildren, or traveling. Who doesn't want that extra spring in their step?

Now, let's not forget about the impact of exercise on your mental well-being. Exercise has been scientifically proven to lift your mood and reduce feelings of anxiety and depression (Robinson et al., 2018). It's an instant refresher for the mind, leaving you refueled and rejuvenated.

So, how do you go about designing an exercise routine that's perfect for you? Well, the key is to start small and gradually build up. Remember, it's not a race—it's about consistency and enjoyment. Here's a simple framework to get you started:

- **Talk to your doctor:** Before starting any new exercise routine, it is crucial to consult your doctor. Your healthcare provider can provide tailored recommendations considering your current health condition and any existing medical issues you may have.

- **Choose things you love:** Exercise can be a delightful experience rather than a tedious task. Whether it's a leisurely walk in the park, a refreshing swim, tending to your garden, or dancing to your favorite tunes, there are numerous enjoyable ways to stay active.

By choosing activities that bring you joy and excitement, you'll find yourself looking forward to moving your body. When you engage in activities that you genuinely love, you're more inclined to maintain a consistent exercise routine.

- **Set achievable goals:** Start with achievable goals that align with your current fitness level. Planning your first marathon wouldn't make sense if you tend to drive a block to the nearest store. Maybe try walking for 20 minutes three times a week or doing a gentle yoga class. As you advance, you can slowly raise the intensity and length of your workouts.

- **Mix it up:** Variety is the spice of life! Incorporate a mix of cardiovascular, strength, and flexibility exercises into your routine. This not only keeps things interesting but also ensures you're reaping the full range of health benefits.

- **Listen to your body:** Pay attention to how your body feels during and after exercise. If something doesn't feel right, don't push through it. It's okay to take a step back and modify your routine as needed.

- **Stay consistent:** Consistency is key when it comes to seeing results. Aim to exercise on most days of the week, but also give yourself permission to rest and recover when necessary.

- **Be informed:** Staying informed about the latest health guidelines, recommendations, new research, developments, and resources concerning aging will always keep you knowledgeable. Power lies within that knowledge.

- **Find a support system:** You can find support in a variety of places. Join a fitness class, ask a friend to be a workout buddy, or simply share your progress with loved ones. Having a support system can help keep you accountable and motivated.

Your goal here is to hit a minimum of 150 minutes of exercise each week if you are over 65. Below is an example of an exercise plan that may be suitable as a starting point (*How Much Physical Activity*, 2023):

Thursday	Saturday	Sunday
Take this day to rest and refuel.	A 30 minute walk.	Use this day to rest and refuel.

Understanding the Role of Nutrition in Overall Well-Being

Nutrition plays a pivotal role in your physical health and energy. Just as you've diligently saved and planned for retirement, investing in your health through a balanced and nutritious diet is equally important.

Picture your body as a finely tuned machine requiring the right fuel to function optimally. A diet rich in essential nutrients provides the foundation for maintaining physical health, boosting energy levels, and supporting your immune system.

Now, let's highlight some key nutrients that are particularly beneficial as we age (*Healthy Meal Planning: Tips for Older Adults*, 2021):

- **Calcium**
  - **Found in:** Dairy products (milk, yogurt, cheese), fortified plant-based milk (soy, almond), leafy greens (kale, spinach), tofu, sardines, salmon.
  - **Importance:** Vital for maintaining bone health and preventing osteoporosis, which becomes more critical as bone density decreases with age.

- **Vitamin D**
  - **Found in:** Fatty fish (salmon, tuna), egg yolks, fortified dairy and plant-based milk, fortified cereals, sunlight exposure.
  - **Importance:** Works in conjunction with calcium to support bone health and aids in the absorption of calcium, particularly important for older adults who may have reduced sun exposure or difficulty synthesizing vitamin D from sunlight.

- **Vitamin B12**

  - **Found in:** Animal products (meat, fish, poultry, dairy), fortified foods (cereals, nutritional yeast), supplements.

  - **Importance:** Essential for nerve function, DNA synthesis, and red blood cell production; deficiencies are common among older adults due to reduced absorption in the gastrointestinal tract.

- **Omega-3 fatty acids**

  - **Found in:** Fatty fish (salmon, mackerel, sardines), walnuts, flaxseeds, chia seeds, hemp seeds.

  - **Importance:** Supports heart health, brain function, and may reduce inflammation, benefiting cognitive function and cardiovascular health in older age.

- **Antioxidants (Vitamin C, Vitamin E, Beta-carotene)**

  - **Found in:** Citrus fruits (oranges, lemons), berries (strawberries, blueberries), nuts and seeds (almonds, sunflower seeds), avocado, spinach, carrots, sweet potatoes.

  - **Importance:** Helps neutralize free radicals, reducing oxidative stress and inflammation associated with aging, and supports immune function and skin health.

- **Fiber**

  - **Found in:** Whole grains (oats, brown rice, quinoa), legumes (beans, lentils), fruits, vegetables, nuts, seeds.

  - **Importance:** Promotes digestive health, regulates blood sugar levels, aids in weight management, and reduces the risk of chronic diseases such as heart disease and diabetes, which become more prevalent with age.

- **Potassium**

  - **Found in:** Bananas, oranges, potatoes, sweet potatoes, tomatoes, spinach, beans, yogurt, fish.

- o **Importance:** Helps regulate blood pressure, maintain proper muscle function, and support heart health, which is especially important for reducing the risk of hypertension and stroke in older adults.

- **Magnesium**
  - o **Found in:** Nuts (almonds, cashews), seeds (pumpkin seeds, sunflower seeds), whole grains, leafy greens (spinach, kale), legumes, dark chocolate.
  - o **Importance:** Plays a role in bone health, muscle function, energy metabolism, and nerve function, with deficiencies potentially contributing to age-related conditions like osteoporosis and muscle weakness.

- **Zinc**
  - o **Found in:** Shellfish (oysters, crab), red meat, poultry, beans, nuts, whole grains, dairy products.
  - o **Importance:** Supports immune function, wound healing, and DNA synthesis, with adequate intake crucial for maintaining overall health and resilience, especially as immune function naturally declines with age.

Now, let's talk practical strategies for incorporating these nutrients into your daily life. Meal planning becomes your secret weapon for success, allowing you to map out nutritious meals for the week ahead. Start by jotting down your favorite recipes and ensuring they include a variety of nutrient-rich ingredients.

When it comes to grocery shopping, aim to fill your cart with colorful fruits and vegetables, lean proteins, whole grains, and healthy fats. Don't forget to read food labels carefully, opting for low-sodium and low-sugar options whenever possible.

As for cooking, embrace the joy of preparing meals from scratch and experimenting with new flavors and culinary techniques. Get creative in the kitchen, involving your loved ones in the cooking process for added enjoyment and connection.

Remember, every bite you take is a step toward a healthier, happier retirement. By prioritizing nutrition and making mindful choices, you're investing in a future brimming with vitality and well-being.

Embrace the power of nutrition as your friend on this remarkable journey. Nourish your body, nurture your soul, and savor each moment of this beautiful chapter called retirement.

Preventing Common Health Conditions Through Proactive Measures

The more that we understand common health conditions, the more prepared we can be to prevent them (Public Health Agency of Canada, 2021):

- **Heart disease**: This silent killer often creeps up unnoticed, but with the right preventive measures, you can significantly reduce your risk. Regular check-ups with your healthcare provider are paramount. Monitoring your blood pressure and cholesterol levels and maintaining a heart-healthy diet rich in fruits, vegetables, and lean proteins can make a world of difference. Incorporating regular exercise into your routine, even if it's just a daily walk, can keep your heart strong and resilient.

- **Diabetes**: As we age, our bodies may become less efficient at processing sugar, increasing the risk of diabetes. By maintaining a healthy weight through balanced nutrition and regular exercise, you can mitigate this risk. Keep an eye on your blood sugar levels through routine screenings and be mindful of your carbohydrate intake. Opt for whole grains, lean proteins, and plenty of fiber to stabilize blood sugar levels.

- **Osteoporosis**: Brittle bones can be a significant concern for retirees, especially women. To fortify your bones and prevent osteoporosis, ensure an adequate intake of calcium and vitamin D through foods like dairy products, leafy greens, and fortified cereals. Strength training exercises like walking, dancing, or yoga help build bone density and strength. Additionally, avoid smoking and limit alcohol consumption, as they can weaken bones over time.

In addition to regular screenings and check-ups, lifestyle changes play a pivotal role in warding off these conditions. Here are a few proactive measures you can implement:

- **Maintain a healthy weight**: Strive for a balanced diet rich in nutrients and portion control. A healthy weight not only reduces the risk of chronic diseases but also enhances overall well-being.

- **Manage stress**: Retirement can bring about significant lifestyle changes, which may sometimes lead to stress. Engage in activities that promote relaxation and stress management, such as meditation, deep breathing exercises, or hobbies you love.

- **Quit smoking**: If you're a smoker, now is the perfect time to kick the habit. Smoking is a leading cause of many chronic diseases and significantly impacts your quality of life. Seek support from healthcare professionals or smoking cessation programs to help you quit for good.

Remember, the key to a fulfilling retirement lies in nurturing your physical, mental, and emotional health. By adopting these proactive measures and embracing a lifestyle that prioritizes well-being, you're giving yourself added years to enjoy the life you've built.

Adapting to Physical Changes and Limitations in Retirement

It's important to acknowledge that along with the newfound freedom or retirement, there may also be physical changes and limitations to navigate. With the right strategies and mindset, you can embrace these changes and continue to lead a fulfilling and active life.

Let's talk about some of the physical changes commonly experienced in retirement. As you age, your body naturally undergoes various transformations. You may notice a decrease in muscle mass, which can lead to feelings of weakness and reduced mobility. Joint stiffness is also a common occurrence, making movement more challenging and uncomfortable. Additionally, changes in metabolism may affect your energy levels and overall health.

Now, here comes the good news: There are plenty of ways to adapt and thrive despite these changes. One of the most effective strategies is incorporating specific exercises into your routine. Exercise not only helps maintain muscle mass and flexibility but also improves mood and overall well-being.

Here are some practical tips for adapting these exercises to accommodate physical changes in retirement (*Aging Changes in the Bones*, 2023):

- **Strength training**: Focus on exercises that target major muscle groups, such as squats, lunges, and resistance band workouts. Strength training helps build and maintain muscle mass, which is crucial for staying active and independent.

- **Flexibility exercises**: Incorporate stretching exercises into your routine to improve joint mobility and reduce stiffness. Yoga and Pilates are excellent options for enhancing flexibility and balance.

- **Low-impact activities**: Consider low-impact exercises such as swimming, cycling, or walking, which are gentle on the joints while still providing significant health benefits.

- **Stay Consistent**: As mentioned above, consistency is key to reaping the full benefits of exercise.

Remember, it's essential to approach exercise with patience and compassion for yourself. You may not be able to do everything you once could, and that's okay. The goal is to stay active and maintain your overall health and well-being.

You can use the exercise program above to build from, and when comfortable, you can begin to add flexibility and strength training exercises.

Adapting to physical changes in retirement is all about embracing a positive mindset and taking proactive steps to maintain your health and vitality. By incorporating exercise into your daily life and listening to your body's needs, you can continue to live life to the fullest in your retirement years.

Prioritizing Adequate Sleep and Managing Stress

We now know that retirement is about nurturing your overall well-being. Two key pillars in this pursuit are prioritizing adequate sleep and managing stress effectively.

Let's start with sleep. In our busy lives, sleep often takes a backseat, but in retirement, you have the opportunity to reclaim your rest. Adequate sleep isn't just about feeling refreshed in the morning; it's about being mindful that nurturing your body, mind, and spirit is essential.

During sleep, your body undergoes essential repair and rejuvenation processes. It's when your brain consolidates memories, your cells regenerate, and your immune system gets a boost. In retirement, you have the luxury of setting your own sleep schedule, so honor your body's natural rhythm. Aim for 7-9 hours of quality sleep each night, and watch how it transforms your days (Mayer, 2021).

Now, let's tackle stress. Retirement doesn't mean you're immune to stress; if anything, it can introduce new sources of tension. Stress can arise from adjusting to newfound freedom, dealing with health concerns, or adjusting to the changes in relationships. It can sneak up on you if left unchecked.

Start by identifying your stressors—what triggers that knot in your stomach or that racing heartbeat? Once you've pinpointed them, devise strategies to tackle them head-on. This might involve practicing mindfulness, engaging in regular exercise, or seeking support from loved ones or professionals.

Remember, stress management isn't about eliminating stress altogether (because, let's face it, some stress is inevitable); it's about building resilience and finding healthy ways to cope. Embrace relaxation techniques like deep breathing, meditation, or spending time in nature. Cultivate hobbies that bring you joy and peace. And don't hesitate to seek guidance if stress becomes overwhelming.

Maintaining an Active and Healthy Lifestyle

Throughout this chapter, we have discussed ways to stay fit and healthy. Most have included exercise routines, but how else can we accomplish this? Consider engaging in activities such as gardening, pickleball, or geocaching. These pursuits not only promote physical activity but also engage your mind and provide a feeling of achievement.

But staying active isn't just about solo pursuits. It's equally important to stay socially connected and engaged. Joining group activities or clubs not only adds variety to your routine but also provides invaluable social support. Whether it's a book club, a hiking group, or a dance class, being part of a community fosters a sense of belonging and strengthens your overall well-being.

Now, let's talk about integrating physical activity into your daily life. Small changes can make a big difference. Instead of taking the elevator, opt for the stairs. Take regular walks in your neighborhood or local park. Even household chores can double up as exercise opportunities. The key is to find ways to keep moving throughout the day, making physical activity a natural part of your lifestyle.

And always keep in mind: It's never too late to begin. Whether you have experience as an athlete or are just starting out, there is something suitable for everyone. Don't be afraid to try new things and step out of your comfort zone.

As you look ahead to the next chapter, get ready to explore the importance of building and nurturing social connections. Just as staying fit enriches your physical well-being, cultivating meaningful relationships is important for your emotional and mental health in retirement.

Get excited to discover practical strategies and empowering advice for creating social networks that bring joy, companionship, and positivity into your life. Together, we'll unlock the secrets to a retirement filled with purpose and lasting happiness.

CHAPTER 6:
BUILDING AND NURTURING
SOCIAL CONNECTIONS

In this chapter, we'll take a positive look at proactive strategies when cultivating strong social bonds and navigating the intricate dance of family dynamics during retirement. Whether you're looking to deepen existing connections or forge new friendships, you'll find practical guidance to help you along the way.

We'll discuss finding a balance between social interactions and personal space, honoring your need for solitude while embracing the joys of companionship. You'll learn how to adapt to changes in family dynamics gracefully, navigating the ebb and flow of relationships with grace and understanding.

Moreover, we'll explore the role of technology in staying connected with loved ones, demystifying the digital landscape to bridge geographical gaps and strengthen ties across generations. Whether it's a video call with a grandchild or sharing memories with friends on social media, technology can be a powerful tool for fostering connection in today's digital age.

Strengthening Existing Relationships and Cultivating New Friendships

Start by valuing the close relationships you have with your family and friends. These connections have been important in your life story. As you retire, it's crucial to nurture these relationships. It's normal to feel a bit unsure during this transition, especially with less daily contact and more free time.

The good news? You can make new connections and prevent loneliness, which can affect your mental well-being. Just like other essential things in life, it takes effort and initiative.

Wondering where to direct your energy? Don't worry; we've got you covered with practical strategies to enrich your social life and nurture meaningful relationships during retirement. Let's dive in (Prvulovic, 2021):

- **Revitalize your relationship:** Inject some spark back into your marriage by dedicating time to date nights. Rather than just going through the motions, explore new retirement activities together. The joy of learning something new as a couple lies in the shared vulnerability. So, why not embark on a new adventure together and rediscover what brought you close in the first place?

- **Share your musical passion:** Pass down your love for music to your grandchildren by teaching them to play an instrument. Alternatively, if music wasn't a big part of your life, why not pick up a new instrument together? Regardless of age, engaging with music stimulates memory and provides a holistic brain workout. Plus, making music together fosters a special bond between grandparents and grandchildren, creating lasting memories.

- **Buddy up for walks:** Boost your mood and prevent chronic diseases by taking daily walks with a friend, neighbor, or family member. Walking is a straightforward yet efficient exercise option suitable for all people. Join a local walking group or initiate walks with friends because it's an opportunity to socialize, stay active, and enjoy the outdoors together.

- **Celebrate family traditions:** Reconnect with your loved ones by initiating or continuing family traditions. Try organizing an annual reunion, sharing your calendar with immediate family, or monthly family meals with extended family. These traditions enhance family connections and form enduring recollections. Focus on activities that resonate with everyone, and cherish the joy of being together.

- **Rediscover romance:** Embrace romance in your senior years to combat loneliness. If you are not married, dating as a mature adult can seem overwhelming. Participating in social activities tailored for older adults or volunteering can expand your social circle and potentially lead to meaningful connections. Remember, nurturing intimacy not only enriches your relationship but also enhances overall well-being.

- **Reconnect with old friends:** Utilize technology to reconnect with old friends and acquaintances. Whether it's a phone call, coffee date, or virtual catch-up, maintaining connections is vital. Reach out to former college buddies, coworkers, or childhood friends—rekindling these relationships brings joy and fulfillment.

- **Foster intergenerational bonds:** As a grandparent, cherish the opportunity to bond with your grandchildren or the children of friends and family. Spending quality time alone with each child fosters unique connections and creates cherished memories. If you don't have grandchildren, consider bonding with young relatives or volunteering with youth organizations to nurture intergenerational relationships.

- **Strengthen sibling connections:** Invest time in deepening your relationship with siblings. Despite life's demands, maintaining a close bond with siblings contributes to reduced loneliness, increased self-esteem, and greater life satisfaction. Regular communication, shared activities, or heartfelt conversations can nurture sibling connections.

- **Engage with extroverts:** Leverage the social prowess of extroverted friends to expand your social circle. Join them in social outings or activities, allowing their outgoing nature to ease any apprehension about meeting new people. Embrace the opportunity to step out of your comfort zone and build meaningful connections.

- **Participate in community activities:** Engage with your local community through religious or spiritual organizations, volunteering, or attending social events. Participating in communal activities fosters a sense of belonging and provides opportunities for social interaction and personal growth. Explore activities aligned with your interests and values to forge genuine connections.

- **Cultivate furry friendships:** If you're a pet owner, capitalize on the opportunity to connect with other pet owners in your neighborhood. Daily walks and visits to dog parks with your furry companion offer opportunities for casual interactions and potential friendships. Embrace the companionship of pets and the social connections they facilitate.

- **Seek support and connection:** Participate in support groups tailored to your experiences and interests. There are groups to help with health challenges, bereavement, or life transitions, and these support groups offer a safe space for sharing experiences and receiving empathy and encouragement. Seek out communities where you feel understood and supported.

Remember, retirement is not synonymous with social isolation. With intentionality and perseverance, you can cultivate a vibrant social life and meaningful relationships in this new chapter of your life.

Overcoming Shyness or Social Anxiety and Initiating Conversations With New People

Retirement opens up a whole new chapter in life, filled with exciting opportunities for personal growth and connection. Yet, it's completely natural to feel a bit nervous about meeting new people or stepping into unfamiliar social situations, especially if you've been out of practice or have struggled with shyness in the past.

First, recognize that feeling shy or anxious in social situations is common and nothing to be ashamed of. Many people experience these feelings to varying degrees, especially when faced with new environments or interactions. The key is not to let these feelings hold you back from embracing the wonderful retirement opportunities. Lean into relaxation techniques such as:

- **Deep breathing:** Slow, deep breaths to calm the mind and body. It focuses on breathing deeply from the diaphragm, which can help reduce stress, promote relaxation, and increase oxygen flow to the brain.

- **Visualization:** Imagine a peaceful, calming scene or a desired outcome. By vividly picturing positive scenarios or experiences, visualization can help reduce anxiety, enhance focus, and promote a sense of well-being.

- **Progressive muscle relaxation:** Systematically tensing and relaxing muscle groups throughout the body. By consciously tensing and then releasing muscle tension, individuals can promote physical relaxation, reduce muscle tension, and alleviate stress and anxiety.

One effective strategy is to shift your focus away from yourself and onto others. Instead of worrying about how you're coming across or what others might think of you, try to genuinely show interest in the people you're interacting with. Ask open-ended questions about their interests, experiences, or opinions. People love to talk about themselves, and by showing curiosity and actively listening, you'll naturally create a more engaging and comfortable conversation environment. Why not try some icebreakers or conversation starters? For example:

Icebreakers or conversation starters can be invaluable for retirees as they navigate social interactions and build connections in their retirement years. Here are some examples tailored for retirees:

- **Memory lane:** Share fond memories from past travels, career highlights, or memorable life experiences.

- **Future dreams:** Encourage discussions about aspirations and goals for the future.

- **Shared interests:** Explore common hobbies or interests that can serve as conversation starters. Maybe gardening, cooking, sports, or arts and crafts? Finding common ground can facilitate meaningful connections.

Another helpful approach is to practice mindfulness and self-compassion. Instead of getting caught up in negative thoughts or self-criticism, try to approach social interactions with kindness and understanding toward yourself. Remind yourself that it's okay to feel nervous and that every interaction is an opportunity for growth and learning.

Additionally, it can be beneficial to gradually expose yourself to social situations that make you feel slightly uncomfortable but not overwhelmingly so. Start by attending small gatherings or events with people you feel comfortable with, and gradually work your way up to larger gatherings or meeting new people one-on-one. Each positive interaction will boost your confidence and help you build momentum toward overcoming your shyness or social anxiety.

Finally, remember to celebrate your successes, no matter how small they may seem. Every time you initiate a conversation with someone new or step outside of your comfort zone, you're taking a courageous step toward personal growth and connection. Be proud of yourself for having the courage to try, and don't be discouraged by setbacks along the way. With patience, persistence, and a positive attitude, your confidence and comfort in social situations will naturally grow over time.

Maintaining a Healthy Balance Between Social Interactions and Personal Space

Social interactions and personal space are both essential for your well-being. Social interactions provide stimulation, support, and connection, while personal space allows you to recharge, reflect, and pursue your individual interests. So, just how do we strike that perfect balance between social interactions and personal space:

- **Recognize Your Needs:**
  - o **Listen to your body and mind:** Pay attention to signals from your body and mind. If you're feeling overwhelmed or fatigued, it may be a sign that you need some personal space to recharge.

o **Allocate "me time" regularly:** Schedule dedicated time for activities you enjoy doing solo. Whether it's reading a book, going for a walk, or indulging in a favorite hobby, prioritize self-care practices that rejuvenate your spirit.

- **Communicate Boundaries:**

    o **Openly discuss your needs:** Have honest conversations with loved ones about your need for personal space. Express your boundaries clearly and respectfully to ensure understanding and support.

    o **Be honest about your needs:** Don't hesitate to communicate what you require to feel balanced and fulfilled. Setting boundaries is essential for maintaining healthy relationships and preserving your well-being.

- **Choose Quality Social Interactions:**

    o **Select activities that align with your interests:** Opt for social engagements that resonate with your passions and values. Whether it's joining a book club, volunteering for a cause you care about, or attending cultural events, prioritize activities that bring joy and fulfillment.

    o **Prioritize meaningful connections:** Focus on nurturing deep, meaningful connections with others rather than spreading yourself too thin with superficial engagements. Quality over quantity is key when it comes to social interactions.

- **Remain Flexible:**

    o **Be open to adjustments:** Recognize that your need for social interactions and personal space may fluctuate over time. Stay flexible and be willing to adapt your balance according to your evolving needs and circumstances.

    o **Understand evolving needs:** As you journey through retirement, understand that your needs and preferences may change. Embrace the process of self-discovery and adjust your balance accordingly.

- **Embrace Positivity:**

  o **Approach retirement with optimism:** Cultivate a positive outlook on retirement, viewing it as a time of opportunity and growth. Embrace the freedom to structure your days in a way that honors both your social and personal needs.

  o **View personal space as vital:** Recognize personal space as a crucial component of overall well-being, essential for self-reflection, relaxation, and pursuing individual interests. Embrace it as a valuable aspect of your retirement lifestyle.

- **Celebrate Your Journey:**

  o **Acknowledge your growth:** Take pride in the progress you've made in finding a balance between social interactions and personal space. Celebrate the positive changes you've implemented in your retirement lifestyle.

  o **Share your experiences:** Use your journey as inspiration to others embarking on their retirement adventure. Share your insights and lessons learned to empower others in crafting fulfilling and balanced retirement lifestyles.

By implementing these strategies, you can cultivate a harmonious balance between social interactions and personal space, fostering a retirement filled with connection, fulfillment, and well-being. Remember, finding balance is an ongoing process, so be patient and compassionate with yourself as you navigate this exciting chapter of life!

Addressing Changes in Family Dynamics and Relationships

Transitioning into retirement opens up a new chapter in life, one where family dynamics and relationships can undergo some shifts. It's a period of adjustment, but with the right mindset and strategies, you can navigate these changes with grace and positivity.

One of the most significant changes you might notice is the newfound amount of time you have to spend with your family. While this can be incredibly rewarding, it can also bring its own set of challenges. Suddenly, having more time together can sometimes highlight differences in expectations, routines, and communication styles.

Another common challenge is finding a new balance between independence and interdependence. After years of working and possibly raising a family, you may find yourself reassessing your roles and responsibilities within your family unit. It's natural to want to maintain your independence and pursue your own interests in retirement, but it's also important to remain connected and supportive of your loved ones.

Additionally, retirement can sometimes bring about changes in power dynamics within the family. As roles shift and responsibilities evolve, it's essential to approach these changes with patience, understanding, and open communication. Your adult children may have grown accustomed to viewing you as the primary decision-maker or provider and adjusting to a more egalitarian relationship can take time and effort from both sides.

Effective Communication Strategies

Even though it's natural for conflicts or shifts in dynamics to arise, the good news is that there are practical steps you can take to navigate these changes with grace and positivity.

- **Active listening:** Focus on fully understanding the speaker's message by giving them your full attention, maintaining eye contact, and providing verbal and nonverbal cues to show that you are engaged and attentive.

- **Empathetic communication:** Seek to understand and acknowledge the emotions and perspectives of others, demonstrating empathy and validation in your responses. Reflecting back on what you've heard and expressing understanding can help build trust and strengthen relationships.

- **Clear and concise messaging:** Communicate your thoughts and ideas clearly and simply, avoiding complicated language or unnecessary details. Organize your message logically to make sure others can easily understand it.

- **Nonverbal communication:** Pay attention to your body language, facial expressions, and tone of voice, as these nonverbal cues can significantly impact how your message is perceived. Maintain open body language, make eye contact, and use a friendly tone to convey warmth and sincerity.

- **Conflict resolution:** Approach conflicts constructively by actively listening to the perspectives of all parties involved, seeking common ground, and collaborating to find mutually acceptable solutions. Use "I" statements to express your feelings and concerns without blaming or criticizing others, and remain calm and respectful during discussions.

Using Technology to Stay Connected

With technology at your fingertips, you can maintain meaningful relationships with family and friends regardless of physical distance.

From video calls to messaging apps, there's a plethora of options available to help you bridge the gap and maintain close connections. Platforms like Zoom, Skype, or FaceTime allow you to see the smiling faces of your loved ones in real-time, no matter where they are in the world. It's like having a virtual coffee date or family reunion right in the comfort of your own home!

But let's not forget about social media. Platforms like Facebook, Instagram, and Twitter aren't just for the younger generation. They're fantastic tools for staying updated on the lives of your loved ones, sharing photos and memories, and even joining interest-based groups or communities where you can connect with like-minded individuals.

And speaking of interests, technology opens up a world of opportunities to explore new hobbies and interests alongside your loved ones. Try joining a virtual book club, taking an online cooking class, or even starting a blog to share your adventures and wisdom with the world; the possibilities are endless.

Overcoming Technological Barriers

Let's acknowledge that technology, for some, can be overwhelming at first, especially if you're not accustomed to it. But it's worth the effort (*Technology for Seniors*, 2023)

- **Start with the basics:** Just like learning any new skill, start with the basics. Familiarize yourself with common devices such as smartphones, tablets, or computers. Experiment with their functions, explore different apps, and don't be afraid to make mistakes. Keep in mind that it's all a component of the learning journey.

- **Seek guidance and support:** Don't hesitate to seek help from family, friends, or even local community centers. Many communities offer technology classes tailored for retirees, where you can learn at your own pace in a supportive environment. Additionally, online tutorials and YouTube videos can be invaluable resources.

- **Stay curious and open-minded:** Approach technology with a curious and open mind. Don't let fear of the unknown hold you back. Embrace the learning process with enthusiasm, knowing that every small step forward is a victory.

- **Practice:** Like any skill, proficiency in technology comes with practice. Make it a habit to use digital devices and platforms regularly. Whether it's sending emails, video calling loved ones, or exploring social media, consistent practice will build your confidence and competence over time.

- **Stay positive and patient:** Be patient with yourself and celebrate your progress, no matter how small. You are not alone on this journey, and each step you take brings you nearer to your goal.

Overcoming technological barriers and learning how to use digital communication effectively is not just about keeping up with the times; it's about embracing new opportunities, staying connected, and enriching your retirement experience. So, seize the moment, embrace the challenge, and let technology be your ally in this exciting chapter of your life!

As we wrap up this chapter on building and nurturing social connections, I hope you're feeling inspired and motivated to enrich your retirement years with vibrant relationships and meaningful connections.

By now, you've learned the importance of fostering social connections in retirement—not just for the enjoyment they bring but also for the numerous benefits they offer. Whether it's spending time with family, reconnecting with old friends, or expanding your social circle through new activities and interests, nurturing these relationships is key to a fulfilling retirement.

As we turn the page to the next chapter, we are going to investigate lifelong learning and continued growth. Retirement isn't a time to stagnate—it's an opportunity to explore new horizons, challenge yourself, and expand that brain.

We'll discover practical strategies for staying intellectually curious, pursuing new hobbies, and embracing personal development in retirement. Get ready to ignite your curiosity, expand your knowledge, and unlock the endless possibilities that retirement has to offer.

CHAPTER 7:
LIFELONG LEARNING AND PERSONAL GROWTH

Are you prepared to awaken your passion for lifelong learning and ongoing development? It's the moment to welcome this new chapter of life with excitement and curiosity, which involves maintaining a sharp mind and an engaged spirit.

Today's retirees are dynamic, vibrant individuals with an insatiable thirst for knowledge and a drive to explore new horizons. In this chapter, we'll enter the wonderful world of lifelong learning, where the benefits are as endless as the opportunities.

We will explore the remarkable impact that ongoing learning can have on your cognitive function, uncovering how it not only enhances your creativity but also boosts your confidence significantly.

Throughout the chapter, you will find strategies to help you get involved in the world of lifelong learning. I invite you to join me on this exhilarating adventure of intellectual growth and personal development. Let's unlock the full potential of your retirement years and make every moment count. The world is waiting, and the possibilities are endless.

Exploring Accessible Educational Programs and Courses for Retirees

For many retirees, returning to school ranks high on their priorities; however, the cost of tuition can be a significant barrier. To support lifelong learning, numerous colleges and universities provide discounted or complimentary college courses for individuals aged 60 and above.

The goal of this section is to place emphasis on the importance of ensuring that retirees can conveniently access lifelong education programs. Regardless of new scheduling conflicts, mobility limitations, or even location, it is imperative that all retirees possess the means to pursue their education effortlessly.

Premier Online Learning Platforms for Senior Learners

As a retiree, continuing your education can be both fulfilling and advantageous. The rapid growth of online learning platforms has made it easier than ever to access quality education from anywhere. According to a 2021 article by ThinkImpact, which compiled data from various e-learning studies, online learning is particularly effective for older adults. Here are some key insights (Roberts, 2022):

- E-learning helps older students retain 25% to 60% more information compared to traditional classroom settings.

- 46% of all students over the age of 60 find online learning to be as effective as face-to-face interaction.

- Since 2020, 98% of universities have offered online courses that retirees can access.

These numbers show how much learning you can do online to gain new skills or knowledge. There are many choices, so first think about how much money you want to invest in your learning, keeping in mind some are free, how much time you can commit, and what subjects you want to learn. Here are nine top online learning sites tailored for older adults (*Top 5 Online Learning Sites for Older Adults*, 2022):

- **Senior Planet:** Senior Planet offers a vast array of courses designed specifically for individuals over 60. Their classes focus on five key areas: social engagement, financial security, health and wellness, civic engagement and advocacy, and creativity. Some popular introductory courses include "Digital Storytelling," "Etsy for Entrepreneurs," "Ready, Set, Bank," and "Fitness Essentials." All live classes are free, making it an excellent resource for those looking to broaden their horizons.

- **U3A:** This acronym stands for The University of the Third Age. In this context, "University" signifies a community of individuals rather than an academic institution. It's about bringing together people who share a passion for a unified set of activities. This initiative is tailored for those in retirement, focusing on lifelong learning and enrichment. It features local learning circles within the community, supplemented by online educational activities and special interest groups. You can discover a new way to enjoy your retirement with a globally wide network of over 1000 groups (What Is the University of the Third Age (U3A)?, n.d.).

- **GetSetUp:** This connects older adults (55+) with peers to learn new skills and unlock life experiences. With a community of over four million learners in 160 countries, they offer live classes, social hours, and special events led by expert instructors. Classes cover diverse topics such as fitness, healthcare, drawing, foreign languages, cooking, music, and business. While there is a free plan with limited access, as of publishing, full access is $19.99 per month, providing entry to over 500 live interactive classes weekly.

- **Full Sail University:** If you are tech-savvy and interested in entertainment, videography, media, visual arts, or communications, Full Sail University might be the right choice for you. This leading creative arts school offers online degree programs designed to provide real-world industry experience and creative problem-solving skills. Their flexible 24/7 e-learning schedule allows you to fit courses into your existing lifestyle. You can see a full list of programs and tuition costs on their website.

- **One Day University:** One Day University offers a unique approach to online learning by partnering with esteemed professors from prestigious universities to deliver their most captivating lectures. You can enjoy live-streamed talks, access hundreds of recorded lectures, and engage in small group discussions with peers. After a free limited trial, access costs $8.99 per month at the time of publishing.

- **BBC Language: A fantastic site where you can learn over** 40 different languages for free! Classes start at the beginner level and move well into advanced. You can join at any level you are comfortable with. As of publishing, the most popular courses are Spanish, German, Italian, and French.

- **Coursera Free:** Don't be surprised when you log in to discover many "paid" options on this site. However, you will notice a selection of courses offered for free. Some of the more popular courses include:

  o Financial Markets

  o Successful Negotiations: Essential Strategies and Skills

  o Financial Engineering and Risk Management

  o Introduction to Philosophy

- **TEDEd:** If you're a retiree, you may be familiar with TEDTalks, a nonprofit lecture series that showcases insights from leading experts worldwide. They now offer a free, new series featuring valuable lessons across various topics, presented in a simple and engaging video format!

- **Academic Earth:** Academic Earth has been providing free online college courses from top universities since 2009. Whether you aim to earn a certificate, a bachelor's degree, or even a doctorate, Academic Earth offers over 60 complete courses in fields such as art, business, engineering, humanities, medicine, science, and math. This platform is ideal for retirees seeking to expand their knowledge at no cost.

For retirees looking to explore online learning, YouTube provides a wide range of global instructors teaching various subjects. You can also access free educational apps like Duolingo, PictureThis, and Brainly on your phone for easy and convenient learning.

Taking Online Classes for Free as a Retiree

Online courses offer a structured environment, which can be particularly beneficial for those adjusting to retirement. Establishing a routine through setting goals, completing assignments, and engaging with course materials can provide a new sense of purpose and accomplishment, significantly enhancing your overall well-being. Additionally, online learning presents an opportunity to discover new interests and passions, making your retirement years even more fulfilling.

Going down the road of lifelong learning is a fulfilling experience, particularly for those who have recently retired. Did you know there are numerous free online degree programs and courses accessible to help you reach your objectives?

Accessing Free Online Courses and Degrees

Options are available for retirees looking to attend college classes without cost. It is important to note that not all paths guarantee a degree. If you want a degree, you should schedule a meeting with an admissions representative to clarify program requirements and any tuition or fees associated with that. Let's break down some ways to achieve free continuing education.

Tuition Waivers

One of the most common ways for retirees to attend college for free is through tuition waiver programs. Many public universities participate in these programs, allowing retirees to enroll without paying tuition. While eligibility requirements vary, some programs are available at two-year colleges offering associate degrees, while others extend to four-year institutions. Typically, the eligibility age ranges from 60 to 65. To take advantage of these opportunities, contact the admissions office of the institution you're interested in to confirm their participation and specific requirements (Scatton, 2023).

Auditing Courses

Another option for seniors is auditing courses, which allow you to attend classes without earning a degree or receiving a grade. Many universities permit students to audit classes that have not reached full enrollment capacity. Although you may not participate in exams or receive a formal grade, auditing is an excellent way to engage with new subjects and stay intellectually active.

Massive Open Online Courses (MOOCs)

Prestigious universities such as Harvard, Yale, the University of Pennsylvania, and Stanford offer MOOCs through platforms like EdX and Coursera. These courses offer a unique opportunity for retirees to learn from esteemed professors and industry experts. While many MOOCs provide a complimentary option with restricted access to materials for a limited time, there is also a paid alternative for those seeking certification upon finishing the course. Though MOOCs generally do not lead to a full degree, they are ideal for upskilling or exploring new subjects (Scatton, 2023).

Senior Discounts

Similar to discounts available at grocery stores and other establishments, retirees can often take advantage of tuition discounts at educational institutions by meeting specific age or income criteria. Furthermore, older learners may also have access to special scholarships, increasing the affordability of higher education for retirees. Don't hesitate to reach out to any institution you are interested in to inquire.

Lifelong learning is a valuable pursuit that can greatly enrich your retirement years. Taking advantage of the various opportunities available allows you to continue to grow intellectually, discover new passions, and maintain a sense of purpose and accomplishment. There are numerous ways to access education and keep your mind engaged regardless of your location or any barriers you might face.

Just like exercising your body keeps it healthy, exercising your brain through learning helps stave off cognitive decline and memory loss. It's like giving your brain a daily workout, keeping it strong and resilient.

How to Choose the Right Learning Avenue in Retirement

Starting down the path of lifelong learning as a retiree is an exciting venture. To ensure you select the most suitable learning avenue, follow these guidelines:

- **Clarify your educational goals:** Start by identifying what you hope to achieve with your education. Are you looking to explore a new interest or deepen your knowledge in a particular area? Understanding your goals will help you focus your search on programs that best suit your aspirations.

- **Review the program's curriculum:** Examine the curriculum of potential programs to ensure they offer courses that align with your interests and goals. Whether you want to learn about art history, digital technology, or environmental science, choosing a program that matches your passions will keep you motivated and engaged.

- **Seek programs tailored to retirees:** Look for online degree programs specifically designed for retirees or older adults. These programs often feature flexible schedules, self-paced learning options, and support services tailored to the needs of mature learners, making it easier to balance education with other retirement activities.

- **Consider accessibility and technology requirements:** Look for programs that are user-friendly and compatible with your devices. Check the accessibility of the platform, the ease of use, and any technological requirements to avoid any unnecessary frustration.

- **Evaluate support services for mature learners:** Strong support services can make your learning experience easier. Look for programs that offer academic advising, tutoring, and access to libraries or research resources. Support services tailored to mature learners can help you navigate any challenges you might face during your studies.

- **Define your educational commitment:** Once you have clarified your educational objectives, decide on the level of commitment you are ready to make. If you aim to explore a new interest, individual courses might be sufficient. However, if you seek a more comprehensive educational experience, consider whether an associate, bachelor's, or master's degree is appropriate and assess the time and effort you can commit to your studies.

Following these steps allows you to choose a learning avenue that not only meets your educational needs but also enriches your retirement years. Lifelong learning can be a rewarding and fulfilling pursuit, offering new knowledge, skills, and experiences that enhance your life in meaningful ways.

Researching Programs

Start your research with online search engines and directories, which can provide valuable information about accredited institutions, tuition costs, and course offerings. Additionally, consulting with academic advisors at colleges or universities can help you understand specific program requirements and course options.

Professional organizations and industry associations are also excellent resources. They can offer insights into the educational requirements for various fields and may have course offerings relevant to your interests.

When you take these steps, you can confidently select a program that meets your needs and supports your lifelong learning journey.

Engaging in educational programs during retirement can also lead to personal growth and fulfillment. It's a chance to challenge yourself and discover new passions and interests. Whether you're learning a new language, mastering a musical instrument, or studying ancient history, each new skill or piece of knowledge adds depth and richness to your life.

Additional Resources

I want to be sure you have all the information possible to set you up for success. Feel free to use the following resources to continue to explore topics to get you excited for lifelong learning.

- **Universities and colleges:** Explore the continuing education departments at nearby universities and colleges. They often offer a variety of courses designed for personal enrichment and skill development.

- **Local recreation centers:** Check with local recreation centers for classes in yoga, painting, photography, and other activities that promote physical and mental well-being. These centers typically provide a welcoming environment for learners of all ages.

- **Adult learning centers:** Some cities have dedicated adult learning centers that offer a range of courses aimed at personal enrichment and skill development. Classes may cover topics like gardening, cooking, finance, and more.

- **Nonprofit organizations:** Investigate nonprofit organizations in your community that focus on education or senior services. They may offer educational opportunities, workshops, or seminars tailored to retirees' interests and needs.

- **Chambers of commerce and cultural centers:** These institutions sometimes collaborate with local businesses and organizations to offer educational events and workshops. These can provide opportunities to learn about local history, business practices, or cultural traditions.

- **Public libraries:** Don't overlook your local public library. Libraries often host author talks, book clubs, lectures, and workshops on a variety of topics. These events are excellent opportunities for engaging in lifelong learning in a familiar and accessible setting.

Essential Tools for Online Learning

To participate in online classes, you will need a few basic items:

- **Computer or device:** Access to the internet is key, and a computer or any device with internet capability is necessary.

- **Internet connection:** A stable internet connection is important, especially for streaming audio and video content.

- **Notebook and pen:** Taking notes can enhance your learning process. While digital tools are available, a traditional notebook and pen can be simpler and more convenient.

- **Headphones:** While optional, headphones can improve your experience, particularly if you have hearing impairments or prefer not to disturb others.

Most retirees already possess these items, eliminating the need for additional expenditures.

In-Person Learning Opportunities

If you prefer in-person learning experiences, consider exploring these local resources:

- **Libraries:** Public libraries are more than just book repositories. Many offer evening and weekend classes on various topics for retirees. Check with your local library for a schedule of available classes.

- **City and county recreation programs:** Local government recreation departments often provide educational programs for seniors. These may include general interest classes as well as those specific to your region, such as local history. Contact your city hall or visit their website to learn about current offerings.

By leveraging these resources, you can continue to pursue knowledge and personal growth, making your retirement years both enriching and enjoyable.

The Power of Online Learning for Retirees

In today's digital era, online learning offers retirees an unparalleled opportunity to engage in lifelong education, broaden their horizons, and enhance their digital proficiency. This modern approach to learning has revolutionized access to information, allowing retirees to explore a wide array of subjects and courses that cater to diverse interests and passions. Let's take a closer look at those now (Wolhuter, 2023):

- **Flexibility and convenience:** Online learning stands out for its remarkable flexibility. Retirees can customize their learning schedules to suit their lifestyles, whether they prefer brief daily sessions or extended study periods. This adaptability ensures that learning becomes an integral, yet manageable, part of their routine.

- **Diverse range of courses:** The variety of courses available online is vast, spanning subjects from the arts and humanities to technology, science, and finance. This extensive selection allows retirees to pursue their interests and explore new areas, fostering a continuous journey of discovery and enrichment.

- **Enhancing digital skills:** Engaging with online learning platforms naturally improves digital literacy. Retirees who may initially feel hesitant about technology can gradually build their proficiency with digital tools, thereby opening new avenues for communication and connectivity.

- **Intellectual stimulation:** Continuous education is crucial for maintaining mental acuity. Online courses provide intellectual challenges that promote critical thinking, problem-solving, and creativity, keeping the mind active and engaged.

- **Connecting with global communities:** Online learning platforms connect learners worldwide. This global interaction allows retirees to engage with diverse perspectives, fostering a sense of global community and broadening their worldviews.

- **Pursuing personal passions:** Retirement presents an ideal opportunity to delve into personal passions. Whether learning a new language, mastering a musical instrument, or studying art history, online learning provides a platform for retirees to explore their curiosities and deepen their interests.

- **Contributing to lifelong fulfillment:** Education is a lifelong journey. Through online learning, retirees can experience a renewed sense of purpose and fulfillment, continuously growing intellectually and embracing new challenges.

- **Boosting confidence:** Mastering new subjects and skills can significantly boost confidence. This newfound self-assurance often extends beyond online learning, positively influencing various aspects of life.

- **Access to renowned instructors:** Many online learning platforms feature courses taught by leading experts. Retirees can benefit from the knowledge and experience of renowned instructors without being limited by geographical boundaries.

- **Expanding social networks:** Online courses encourage interaction and collaboration with other learners. Participating in discussions and group projects fosters social connections, reduces feelings of isolation, and enhances overall well-being.

Embracing lifelong learning through online education is a transformative choice for retirees. It enables intellectual stimulation, skill enhancement, and the pursuit of personal passions. The flexibility and convenience of online courses make them accessible to everyone, regardless of location or age. By exploring a diverse range of subjects, connecting with global communities, and learning from esteemed instructors, retirees can enrich their lives and continue to grow in their retirement years.

Engaging in and Discussing the Benefits of Intellectual Pursuits and Expanding Knowledge

It's more than just keeping your brain in tip-top shape; it's also about feeding your soul. Retirement is the perfect time to explore subjects that have always intrigued you or to delve into entirely new areas of interest. If you have always wanted to learn more about the solar system, horticulture, or literature, now is your chance to immerse yourself fully.

Reading is one of the most accessible and enjoyable ways to expand your knowledge during retirement. Whether you prefer fiction or non-fiction, there's a vast universe of books waiting to be discovered. Not only does reading expose you to new ideas and perspectives, but it also provides a wonderful escape from the everyday stresses of life.

Attending lectures or workshops is another fantastic way to broaden your horizons. Many online classes cover a wide range of topics, from philosophy to technology to gardening, giving you the opportunity to learn from experts in their fields and connect with like-minded individuals.

And let's not forget the power of discussion groups and book clubs. Engaging in thoughtful conversations with others who share your interests can be incredibly stimulating and rewarding. Not only do these interactions provide social connection, but they also offer the chance to deepen your understanding of the subjects you're passionate about.

Embracing Curiosity and a Growth Mindset

Curiosity—the spark that ignites the fire of your passion for life. Curiosity is what keeps us engaged, excited, and eager to explore the world around us. As you enter retirement, it's crucial to nurture and cultivate this curiosity within yourself. You can accomplish this by picking up a new hobby, learning to cook some new recipes, traveling to new places, or simply exploring different cultures, let your curiosity be your guide.

Now, let's pair that curiosity with a growth mindset. This mindset is all about believing in your ability to learn, grow, and adapt to new challenges. Instead of seeing retirement as a time to coast, view it as an opportunity for personal development and self-improvement. By adopting a growth mindset, you'll be more open to trying new things, taking risks, and pushing past the everyday.

Why is this so important? Well, for starters, maintaining mental agility is key to staying sharp and engaged as you age. By challenging yourself with new experiences and learning opportunities, you're essentially giving your brain a workout, keeping it healthy and resilient. Plus, staying open to new challenges and experiences can give you a renewed sense of purpose and fulfillment during retirement.

So, how can you put this into action? Start by identifying areas of interest or curiosity that you've always wanted to explore. Is there a vacation spot you always wanted to explore? A class you have been putting off? A new dish you've wanted to attempt? Maybe you've been toying with the idea of starting your own business? Whatever it is, make a commitment to yourself to pursue it wholeheartedly.

Next, adopt a growth mindset by reframing any challenges or setbacks as opportunities for learning and growth. Instead of getting discouraged, ask yourself, "What can I learn from this?" or "How can I use this experience to become better?"

Finally, surround yourself with people who inspire and support your journey of curiosity and growth. Join clubs, classes, or groups where you can connect with like-minded individuals who share your interests and passions. Make sure there are people within your circle you can continue to learn from and lean on.

Recognizing the Importance of Continued Mental Stimulation

I want you to picture your brain as a muscle. Just like your biceps or your abs, it needs regular exercise to stay strong and resilient. Without that stimulation, it can start to atrophy, leading to cognitive decline and even serious conditions like dementia.

There are countless ways to keep your mental gears turning in retirement! Let's start with puzzles. Whether it's a crossword, Sudoku, or a jigsaw, puzzles are like a workout for your brain. They challenge your problem-solving skills, boost your memory, and keep those neurons firing on all cylinders. Plus, they're a lot of fun!

Then there are brain-training exercises. Thanks to modern technology, you can now access a whole world of apps and games designed to keep your mind agile. From memory games to logic puzzles, these exercises are like a personal trainer for your brain, helping you stay sharp and focused. Go to the Apple or Play Store app on your phone and search "brain training apps," and voila!

Throughout these chapters, we have discussed the importance of social interaction in cognitive function. Studies have shown that staying socially engaged can have a profound impact (Piolatto et al., 2022). So, make it a point to stay connected with friends, join clubs or community groups, or keep volunteering. You will be stimulating your mind and building meaningful connections throughout the process.

Ultimately, your goal should be to embrace curiosity, stay open to new experiences, and never stop learning. So go ahead, challenge yourself, try new things, and keep your mind as vibrant and alive as ever. Your brain keeps thanking you for it!

By embracing the pursuit of knowledge and personal development, you've taken a powerful step toward ensuring your retirement years are as fulfilling as possible. But remember, the journey to happiness and fulfillment is ongoing, and there's always more to discover, learn, and experience.

As you've learned, retirement is about seizing the opportunity to explore new interests, develop new skills, and expand your horizons. Maybe you're learning a new language, taking up a hobby you've always been curious about, or diving into subjects that ignite your passion. Each new endeavor enriches your life in ways you may never have imagined.

However, the benefits of lifelong learning extend beyond personal growth. As you continue to cultivate your mind and broaden your perspectives, you also open yourself up to new opportunities for connection and contribution. And that's where the next chapter comes in: giving back through volunteering and philanthropy.

As you transition into this next phase of your retirement, remember that giving back isn't just about making a difference in the lives of others—it's also about finding deeper meaning and purpose in your own life.

So, as you close this chapter and prepare to start the next leg of your retirement adventure, I encourage you to keep an open mind, embrace new opportunities, and continue to pursue growth and learning with enthusiasm and curiosity. And remember, the best is yet to come!

CHAPTER 8:
GIVING BACK: VOLUNTEERING AND PHILANTHROPY

As you move through retirement, you'll find that it's not just about basking in the warmth of leisure; it's about infusing each day with purpose and meaning. And what better way to do that than by extending a helping hand to others through volunteer work and philanthropy?

In this chapter, we're discovering the transformative power of giving back. We'll explore how volunteering and philanthropy can be the cornerstone of a fulfilling retirement, enriching your life in ways you never imagined. It's not just about what you can give to others; it's about what you receive in return—a sense of purpose, connection, and profound satisfaction.

As a retiree, you possess a treasure trove of wisdom, skills, and experiences garnered over a lifetime. And now is the perfect time to share that wealth with your community. You can consider mentoring young minds, lending a hand at a local shelter, or supporting a cause close to your heart. There are countless opportunities for you to make a tangible difference.

But giving back isn't just about altruism; it's also a powerful catalyst for personal growth and fulfillment. As you engage in volunteer work and philanthropy, you'll discover new passions, forge meaningful connections, and reignite your sense of purpose. Each act of kindness ripples outward, creating a ripple effect of positivity that touches not only the lives of others but also your own.

Throughout this chapter, we'll uncover practical strategies and insights to help you start giving back. From finding the right volunteer opportunities to navigating the world of philanthropy, I'll equip you with the tools and inspiration you need to make a meaningful impact.

Finding Volunteer Opportunities That Align With Personal Interests and Values

Identifying volunteer opportunities that align with your interests and values is vital. Think about the activities that truly ignite your passion. What causes or issues have always resonated with you? Whether it's working with children, caring for animals, preserving the environment, or supporting the elderly, there's bound to be something out there that speaks to your heart.

Consider your skills and expertise accumulated over a lifetime. What talents do you possess that could serve others? Perhaps you have a knack for teaching, organizing events, or even just lending a compassionate ear. Your unique set of skills can make a significant difference in the lives of those you choose to help.

Moreover, don't underestimate the importance of finding volunteer opportunities that resonate with your values. When you align your actions with your deeply held beliefs, you not only make a positive impact on the world but also experience a profound sense of fulfillment and satisfaction.

More than one out of every five older adults volunteer, and it's a great thing to do. Volunteering is a meaningful opportunity for people of all ages, but it's especially beneficial for retirees. A study in the Australian Journal of Psychology in 2019 discovered that the more people volunteer, the happier they tend to be (Lagemann, 2022).

Let's have a closer look at some strategies you can use to maximize your efforts and energy to give back to others and their community.

Research shines a spotlight on the remarkable rewards waiting for those who volunteer regularly. Just a modest commitment of around two hours per week can total 100 hours a year over four years and can lead to so many advantages (Lagemann, 2022):

- **Live longer:** Yes, volunteering can literally add more years to your life!

- **Improved physical abilities:** Say goodbye to limitations and hello to a more active lifestyle.

- **Enhanced mental and emotional wellness:** Dive into a sea of optimism and purpose, fostering a deeper connection to life's joys.

Volunteering shows that you still have time and skills to offer. It's a chance to continue your career in a new way. Enter this next phase confidently, knowing your efforts are appreciated, and your skills are needed.

As you get ready to start volunteering, consider this advice:

- **Trust your instincts:** If something doesn't feel right, trust your gut and explore other opportunities.

- **Seek reputable organizations:** Platforms like volunteermatch.org or idealist.org can help you find trustworthy volunteering opportunities.

- **Prioritize your well-being:** Your health and happiness come first. Ensure the organizations you choose align with your values and treat volunteers with respect.

Now, onto the fun part—choosing the perfect volunteering opportunity for you! Whether you're passionate about mentoring, nurturing, or getting your hands dirty, there's something out there tailored just for you. Here are some ideas to ignite your imagination:

- **Local charities:** Have a look into your community's needs by supporting organizations like Habitat for Humanity, Feeding America, or the Alzheimer's Association.

- **National parks:** If you love the great outdoors, consider lending a hand at local, state, or national parks, engaging in tasks from nature conservation to visitor guidance.

- **Meals on Wheels:** Join the mission of delivering essential nutrition to older adults in your community, making a tangible difference in their lives.

- **Animal shelters:** Show some love to our furry friends by volunteering at your local animal shelter, whether it's providing care or advocating for animal rights.

- **Foster grandparent programs:** There is a great need for youth who don't have grandparents available to them. Share your wisdom and kindness with children in need, leaving a lasting impact on their lives.

- **Community gardens:** Cultivate both plants and connections in your local community garden, sharing your passion for gardening with others.

- **School support:** Support the next generation by volunteering in schools, whether it's tutoring, assisting teachers, or chaperoning field trips.

- **Cuddle programs:** Were you aware that many local children's hospitals have a need that you could fill in their children's ward? Babies who are born premature benefit greatly from cuddles, and their parents can't always be there 24/7. Join a cuddle program and offer cozy snuggles for those wee ones.

Remember, the key is to choose something that sparks joy and aligns with your interests and schedule.

The Impact of Philanthropy on Personal Fulfillment and Well-Being

Retirement marks a new chapter in life, one where you have the opportunity to explore passions and interests and perhaps even fulfill a long-held desire to give back to your community or the world at large. Philanthropy isn't just about donating money; it's about contributing your time, skills, and resources to make a positive difference, and the benefits are truly remarkable.

Engaging in philanthropic activities during retirement offers a profound sense of purpose. After years of dedicated work in your career, you may find yourself seeking a deeper meaning, something that transcends the daily grind. By getting involved in causes you care about, you're aligning your actions with your values. This alignment creates a powerful sense of purpose that can be incredibly fulfilling.

Moreover, the act of giving back instills a profound sense of satisfaction and fulfillment. There's something truly special about knowing that your actions, no matter how small they may seem, are making a positive impact on the lives of others. Maybe you want to help feed the homeless, support educational initiatives, or care for the environment. Each contribution adds up to create meaningful change. This sense of fulfillment is invaluable, contributing to a deep sense of contentment and happiness in retirement.

However, the benefits of philanthropy extend beyond personal fulfillment. Numerous studies have shown a strong correlation between engaging in charitable activities and improved mental well-being. When we give back, our brains release feel-good chemicals like dopamine and oxytocin, often referred to as the "helper's high." These chemicals not only boost your mood but also reduce stress and anxiety, leading to overall better mental health (Breeding, 2020).

Furthermore, philanthropy fosters a sense of connectedness and belonging. In retirement, it's easy to feel disconnected from the world, especially if you're no longer part of a traditional work environment. By getting involved in philanthropic endeavors, you're joining a community of like-minded people who share your passion for making a difference.

Creating a Legacy Through Charitable Contributions

As you transition into retirement, you have the opportunity to leave a lasting impact on the world, one that extends far beyond your lifetime. By making meaningful charitable contributions, you have the power to make a difference in the lives of others, leaving behind a legacy that reflects your values and passions.

It's not just about the financial aspect; it's about making a genuine difference in the lives of those in need. For example, you may choose to support education, healthcare, environmental conservation, or any other cause close to your heart. Your contributions can create ripple effects of positivity that resonate for generations to come.

Now, let's explore the various ways you can contribute. Financial donations are perhaps the most straightforward method, where you can provide direct support to organizations and initiatives that align with your values. You could donate a one-time gift or regular contributions, every dollar counts and can make a significant impact.

Endowments offer another avenue for leaving a lasting legacy. By establishing an endowment, you can ensure sustained support for a cause you're passionate about, even after you're no longer here. Endowments provide a perpetual source of funding, enabling organizations to continue their vital work indefinitely.

Establishing a charitable foundation can be incredibly rewarding for those seeking a more hands-on approach. This allows you to actively make decisions and direct funds toward specific projects or initiatives. With your guidance, your foundation can become a source of hope and support for causes dear to your heart.

Remember, the key to creating a meaningful legacy through charitable contributions lies in aligning your giving with your values and passions and identifying your impact goals. Take the time to reflect on what matters most to you and explore opportunities to make a difference in those areas. Whether you're supporting local initiatives or global causes, your contributions have the power to transform lives and leave a legacy of kindness and compassion.

Seize the opportunity to create a legacy that transcends generations through charitable contributions. By giving back to causes you believe in, you can leave behind a legacy of positivity, compassion, and hope. Your contributions, no matter how big or small, have the power to make the world a better place for years to come.

Those Who Created a Legacy Through Philanthropic Efforts

The Rockefellers

For the Rockefellers, the spirit of giving runs deep within their family veins, shaping their values across generations. Their legacy spans three centuries, highlighting their enduring commitment to making a positive impact on the world.

At the heart of their philanthropy is the belief that wealth brings with it a profound responsibility to uplift others. This principle, instilled by earlier generations, continues to guide the philanthropic endeavors of the Rockefellers today, influencing their priorities and perspectives on giving.

Their journey starts with John D. Rockefeller, Sr. (JDR). He inherited his father's business sense and his mother's kindness. Growing up, he learned the value of giving back, which he embraced throughout his life, even when he was earning only $45 a year. (*The Rockefellers: A Legacy of Giving*, 2017).

As JDR became highly successful in the petroleum industry through the establishment of Standard Oil, he realized he could use his wealth not only to make money but also to benefit society. In addition to investing in different industries, he also donated a large part of his fortune to charitable endeavors (*The Rockefellers: A Legacy of Giving*, 2017).

JDR started giving back in the mid-19th century and later created the Rockefeller Foundation in the early 20th century. He began by helping people and organizations linked to the Baptist church and education, but then he started focusing on bigger social problems. Through programs that support medical education, public health, and labor relations, the Rockefeller Foundation has been a leader in impactful charitable work. This legacy continues through seven generations of Rockefellers, who proudly continue the family's tradition (*The Rockefellers: A Legacy of Giving*, 2017).

Today, with more than 150 descendants of John D. Rockefeller, Sr., the Rockefellers are still actively involved in philanthropy, creating new and effective ways to tackle the world's biggest problems. Their journey showcases how generosity can make a lasting impact, highlighting a united family's significant influence when dedicated to creating positive change (*The Rockefellers: A Legacy of Giving*, 2017).

Andrew Carnegie

Andrew Carnegie, a wealthy and influential figure in the late 1800s and early 1900s, was famous not only for his riches but also for his significant charitable contributions. He started as a messenger in 1835 for a telegraph company and worked hard to advance, eventually becoming a leader at the Pennsylvania Railroad in his mid-twenties (*Andrew Carnegie's Story*, 2019).

But Carnegie didn't stop with his ambitions. He explored different business interests, such as railways and steel production, and became one of the most successful entrepreneurs of his time. Carnegie strongly believed in giving back to society despite his focus on business.

His journey of giving back started in the 1870s when he began building free public libraries in his hometown of Dunfermline. Over time, this effort expanded globally. His marriage to Louise Whitfield further strengthened his dedication to helping others, as they promised to donate most of their wealth while they were alive. Carnegie believed that wealthy people should help others by using their money for good. He practiced what he preached by selling his steel company for a huge amount and giving away his wealth to help others (*Andrew Carnegie's Story*, 2019).

Through his generosity, Carnegie made a lasting impact on the world. He funded libraries, churches, colleges, and nonprofit organizations, shaping communities and improving lives for future generations. His legacy continues through trusts and institutions that carry his name, all of which work to promote education, science, and peace (*Andrew Carnegie's Story*, 2019).

Today, we can draw inspiration from Andrew Carnegie's remarkable story. His journey from humble beginnings to global philanthropist serves as a testament to the power of vision, hard work, and generosity.

As retirees, we, too, have the opportunity to leave a lasting legacy through financial means and our time, wisdom, and compassion. Let's embrace the giving spirit of Carnegie and Rockefeller and make a positive impact in our communities, ensuring that our legacy of kindness and generosity endures for future generations to come.

Offering Skills and Expertise to Support Community Organizations

Think about all the knowledge and experience you've amassed throughout your career. You've likely honed skills that are invaluable to nonprofits and other community groups. Maybe you're an expert in finance, marketing, event planning, or project management. There's a place for you to lend your talents.

Here's how you can get started:

- **Identify your passion:** Reflect on the causes and issues that resonate with you. Is there a particular nonprofit organization or community group whose mission aligns with your values? Start by researching local organizations and finding one that speaks to your heart.

- **Reach out:** Once you've identified a few organizations of interest, reach out to them! Many nonprofits are in constant need of volunteers with specialized skills. Offer your expertise and let them know how you can contribute. Whether it's helping with financial planning, designing marketing materials, or providing strategic advice, your skills can make a world of difference.

- **Mentorship opportunities:** Another fantastic way to utilize your professional expertise is by mentoring younger generations. Consider volunteering as a mentor for students, recent graduates, or aspiring professionals in your field. Your guidance and wisdom can be incredibly valuable as they navigate their own career paths.

- **Join advisory boards:** Many nonprofits have advisory boards comprised of experienced professionals who provide guidance and strategic direction. Consider joining such a board where you can lend your expertise to help steer the organization toward success.

- **Offer workshops or training:** Leverage your expertise by offering workshops or training sessions for members of the community. Whether it's teaching financial literacy, leadership skills, or career development workshops, your knowledge can empower others to succeed.

Remember, by contributing your skills and expertise to support community organizations, you're not just giving back—you're also enriching your own life in profound ways. The sense of fulfillment that comes from making a positive impact is truly unparalleled. So, embrace this new chapter of your life with enthusiasm and know that your contributions are making a difference, one skill at a time!

Real Retired Professionals Who Contribute Their Expertise

Brad the Contractor

Meet Brad, a retired contractor who has woven his passion for construction into a remarkable journey of giving back to his community. From his humble beginnings fetching materials on job sites to mastering the craft and running his own successful company, Brad's career in construction was both physically demanding and immensely satisfying.

Retirement, however, posed a challenge for Brad. After spending decades building homes and structures, the idea of stepping away from work left him feeling adrift. Sure, there were always tasks around the house to tackle, but Brad found himself craving something more meaningful, something that tapped into his expertise and allowed him to make a difference.

It was during those early years of retirement that Brad's friend approached him with an opportunity to get involved with Habitat for Humanity, an organization dedicated to providing homes for families in need. Instantly, Brad felt a spark reignite within him. Here was a chance to not only utilize his skills but also to contribute to a cause he deeply believed in.

Without hesitation, Brad dove into the world of volunteering. He showed up on-site, ready to lend a hand wherever it was needed. Whether it was swinging a hammer, coordinating teams, or offering guidance to fellow volunteers, Brad threw himself into every task with enthusiasm and dedication.

As time went on, Brad's involvement with Habitat for Humanity only deepened. What started as a simple offer to help out transformed into a regular commitment of three days a week. Brad became a cornerstone of the organization, using his experience and leadership to spearhead projects and make a tangible impact on the lives of families in his community.

But Brad's generosity didn't stop there. Motivated by the desire to do even more, he established his own fund to support Habitat for Humanity's mission. Every year, Brad's fund helps to provide a home for a family in need, ensuring that his legacy of giving back will continue long into the future.

Kathy and her Knitting Needles

Kathy had been a dedicated nurse whose passion for caring knew no bounds. For 42 years, she poured her heart and soul into her profession, nurturing patients back to health and bringing comfort to those in need. Nursing wasn't just a job for Kathy; it was her calling, the very essence of who she was.

But as fate would have it, health issues forced Kathy to retire earlier than she had planned. Suddenly, the bustling hospital corridors she once navigated with ease became a distant memory, replaced by the quiet solitude of retirement. Without the constant rhythm of her work, Kathy found herself adrift, her body weary from years of long shifts, her spirit dimmed by the sudden void in her life.

For a while, Kathy withdrew from the world, cocooning herself in loneliness and sadness. The thought of venturing out into a new chapter of life seemed daunting, and she struggled to find purpose in her newfound freedom.

Then, one fateful day, a simple visit to the hospital reignited a spark within Kathy's soul. As she wandered the familiar halls, she stumbled upon a group of volunteers knitting tiny hats and blankets for newborns in the NICU. Intrigued, Kathy struck up a conversation with one of the volunteers and learned about their mission to provide warmth and comfort to premature babies and their families.

In that moment, something stirred inside Kathy—a sense of purpose, a glimmer of hope. She realized that retirement wasn't just about stepping back; it was about finding new ways to give back and make a difference in the lives of others.

With determination in her heart and colorful wool in hand, Kathy set out to knit beautiful blankets and hats for the tiniest patients in need. Each stitch was infused with love and care, a testament to her unwavering dedication to healing, even in retirement.

And as word spread of Kathy's kindness, so did the need for her talents. Before long, she found herself dedicating her mornings to knitting for cancer patients undergoing chemotherapy, bringing warmth and comfort to those facing their own battles.

Today, Kathy's days are filled with purpose and joy, her hands busy creating comfort for those in need. Retirement may have taken her from the hospital floor, but it could never extinguish the light of compassion that burns bright within her.

Kathy's story is a reminder that retirement is an opportunity to channel our skills and talents into acts of kindness that ripple far beyond ourselves. And in giving back to our communities, we find fulfillment, purpose, and the true essence of what it means to live a life of meaning.

Volunteering and philanthropy are not just activities; they're expressions of compassion, generosity, and empathy. They allow you to connect with your community, forge meaningful relationships, and leave a lasting legacy that transcends material wealth.

As we transition into the final chapter of your retirement adventure, let's carry forward the lessons we've learned about the importance of giving back and apply them to the next phase: embracing travel and adventure. Just as volunteering and philanthropy enrich our lives, so too can exploration and discovery ignite our spirits and broaden our horizons.

In the chapters ahead, we'll delve into the transformative power of travel, the joys of exploring new cultures, and the thrill of embarking on adventures both near and far. Get ready to pack your bags, open your heart to new experiences, and savor every moment of this remarkable phase of life they call retirement.

CHAPTER 9:
EMBRACING TRAVEL AND ADVENTURE

You've journeyed through eight of the habits of a happy retiree, and now it's time to explore the last and what some consider the most exhilarating aspects of retirement: travel and adventure. In this final chapter, we're going to dive deep into the world of exploration, discovery, and limitless possibilities that await you.

Travel and adventure are not just about ticking off destinations on a bucket list. They're about embracing the unknown, opening yourself up to new experiences, and immersing yourself in different cultures and landscapes. They're about discovering the world outside your comfort zone and finding joy, enrichment, and personal growth along the way.

But I understand that the idea of travel and adventure can sometimes be daunting, especially if you're stepping into retirement with apprehension or uncertainty. That's why this chapter is here to guide you, to provide you with practical strategies and advice to help you navigate the exciting world of travel and adventure with confidence and enthusiasm.

And remember, travel and adventure are not just for the young or the physically fit. No matter your age or physical ability, there are opportunities for exploration and discovery waiting for you. So don't let fear or hesitation hold you back. Embrace the unknown, step outside your comfort zone, and let the journey of a lifetime begin. After all, the world is waiting, and your adventure starts now.

Planning and Preparing for Travel Experiences

The possibilities for travel in retirement are as endless as your imagination! As you step into this new phase of life, filled with freedom and extra time, crafting the perfect travel bucket list becomes a thrilling adventure in itself. Let's look at some practical strategies and insightful advice to make your travel dreams a reality.

- **Assess your health and fitness:** Age is just a number, and many retirees show that life can be exciting and full of activity even in their 90s. When planning your travels, it's important to think about your health, fitness, and mobility. First, assess your abilities realistically, including stamina, mobility, and cognitive sharpness. Plan your trips according to how physically demanding they are. Start with more adventurous journeys at the beginning of retirement and move toward easier explorations as you get older.

  o Take into account factors like time zone changes, flight durations, walking requirements, and accessibility.

  o Be realistic about your capabilities to ensure a fulfilling and enjoyable travel experience.

  o Remember, it's not about limitations—it's about adapting and embracing new adventures at every stage of life.

- **Plan multi-generational adventures:** Traveling with family creates special memories that last for many years. Try spending time with grandchildren or discovering new places with grown-up children.

- Trips with different generations provide chances for bonding and making memories together.

  o Take advantage of concierge services and travel planners to organize activities suitable for all ages.

  o Embrace the support and companionship of family members during your travels.

  o Create lasting memories that transcend age barriers and strengthen family bonds.

- **Don't wait; start today:** Time is a precious gift, and there's no better moment to start your travel adventures than now. Maybe you want to plan a grand expedition or a spontaneous weekend getaway. Every travel experience enriches your life in remarkable ways, so get planning!

- o Embrace the spontaneity of travel and seize every opportunity to explore new destinations.

- o Cherish each moment and create a lifetime of unforgettable experiences.

- o Remember, the world awaits—start your adventure today!

As you step into retirement, you should explore the wonderful world of travel. One crucial aspect to consider is how you can plan and prepare for unforgettable experiences, starting with creating a well-thought-out travel budget.

Creating a travel budget:

- Did you know that according to a recent survey, retirees spend an average of 10-20% of their annual income on travel (Rosenberg, 2024)? It's essential to assess your finances and determine a realistic travel budget that aligns with your retirement income.

- Start by listing your desired destinations and estimating the cost of transportation, accommodation, meals, activities, and incidentals.

- Consider setting aside a separate travel fund or allocating a portion of your retirement savings specifically for travel expenses.

Researching destinations and accommodations:

- With endless travel options available, take the time to research destinations that match your interests, preferences, and budget.

- Utilize online resources, travel guides, and recommendations from friends and family to gather information about attractions, local culture, and safety.

- When selecting accommodations, consider factors such as location, amenities, reviews, and accessibility. Whether you prefer luxury resorts, cozy bed and breakfasts, or adventurous camping, there's something for everyone!

Health and safety factors:

- Prioritize your health and safety by considering any medical conditions, dietary restrictions, or mobility concerns when planning your travels.

- Consult with your healthcare provider to ensure you're up-to-date on vaccinations and medications, especially if you're traveling abroad.

- Research healthcare options and emergency services available at your destination, and purchase travel insurance for added peace of mind.

Making necessary arrangements:

- Organize your travel documents well in advance, including passports, visas, driver's licenses, and any required permits or reservations.

- Check for travel advisories and stay informed about local regulations, weather conditions, and potential risks.

- Invest in travel insurance to protect yourself against unforeseen circumstances such as trip cancellations, medical emergencies, or lost luggage.

Remember, retirement is your time to thrive and indulge in the joys of travel. You'll embark on unforgettable adventures with confidence and enthusiasm by implementing these practical strategies and taking proactive steps to plan and prepare.

Exploring Different Types of Travel and Adventure Activities

Embarking on thrilling travel and adventure escapades is a huge bonus of retirement.

Let's explore a myriad of options that promise to infuse your retirement years with a burst of excitement:

- **Eco-tourism:**
  - Immerse yourself in the wonders of nature while also contributing to conservation efforts.
  - Explore biodiverse regions such as the Amazon rainforest, the Galapagos Islands, or the Serengeti.
  - Engage in activities like wildlife spotting, bird watching, or sustainable hiking tours.
  - Visit a sea turtle conservation project in Costa Rica or Mexico. Feel a profound connection with nature and make a positive impact on the environment.

- **Cultural immersion:**
  - Immerse yourself in rich cultures around the globe.
  - Live like a local by staying in homestays or small guesthouses.
  - Participate in cultural workshops, cooking classes, or traditional ceremonies.
  - If time and money allow, spend a month in a small village in Vietnam, learning the language, traditions, and cuisine and forging lasting friendships with the locals.

- **Adventure sports:**
  - Embrace your adventurous spirit with adrenaline-pumping activities.
  - Try your hand at activities like scuba diving, kayaking, or white-water rafting for the really brave.

- o Explore destinations renowned for adventure sports, like New Zealand, Switzerland, or Costa Rica.

- o Real-life example: Mark, at the age of 65, fulfilled his lifelong dream of scuba diving in the Great Barrier Reef, feeling a sense of liberation and exhilaration like never before.

- **Volunteer tourism:**

  - o Make a meaningful difference while exploring new places.

  - o Volunteer for causes close to your heart, such as education, healthcare, or community development.

  - o Engage with local communities and leave a positive impact on their lives.

  - o Real-life example: Lisa dedicated part of her travel during retirement to volunteer teaching English in rural schools across Southeast Asia, finding immense fulfillment in empowering young minds and fostering cross-cultural understanding.

- **Group travel:**

  - o Share your adventures with like-minded individuals and forge new friendships.

  - o Join group tours tailored for retirees to explore destinations hassle-free.

  - o Enjoy the camaraderie of group activities while still having the freedom to explore independently.

- **Travel in your own backyard:**

  - o Take advantage of this time to explore the country you live in. Research those places you have always wanted to visit.

  - o Rent an RV and tour the coast. Make unplanned stops at local restaurants and beaches.

  - o Pack up the camping gear and hit up the National Parks. Soak up the outdoor air and say hello to Mother Nature.

Remember, retirement is your chance to write the next chapter of your life, filled with adventure, exploration, and endless possibilities. So, dare to step out of your comfort zone, embrace the unknown, and let the world be your playground. Your retirement years are waiting to be filled with unforgettable experiences and meaningful connections.

Solo Travel for Retirees

Solo travel in retirement might not have been on your radar earlier in life, but trust me, it's a game-changer. It's a chance to relaunch your life with a burst of energy and excitement that you may not have experienced before. Think of it as a journey of self-discovery and personal growth.

Now, let's address some important points about solo travel during retirement. First, it's all about you—your interests, your agenda, your timetable. No more worrying about meeting the demands of others or sticking to someone else's schedule. Solo travel allows you to march to the beat of your own drum and rediscover your natural rhythm.

As you embark on this adventure, you'll learn so much about yourself. It's not just about the places you visit; it's about the journey within. Solo travelers in their golden years often radiate a joy for life that's infectious. They've embraced the freedom to explore and live life on their terms.

Now, let's talk about the exciting new opportunities awaiting you as a solo traveler in retirement. Forget what you knew about travel back in the day. The landscape has evolved, offering a plethora of options to suit every taste and preference.

Gone are the days of limited choices between independent travel and bus tours. Today, you have a smorgasbord of options, from curated small-group tours to river cruises and everything in between. And yes, solo travel doesn't mean roughing it out in hostels anymore. Luxury hostels with single rooms and vibrant social scenes are now the norm.

Technology has revolutionized the way we travel, offering enhanced safety and connectivity. With just a smartphone and a data plan, you can stay connected with loved ones back home, access vital information, and navigate unfamiliar terrain with ease.

But within the excitement, it's essential to prioritize your destinations wisely. Choose places that truly speak to your soul, where you can immerse yourself in your passions and interests. And remember, it's okay to feel a little stressed at times. Knowing how you respond to stress can help you move through challenging situations with grace and resilience.

Consider blending different travel styles to create a unique experience that suits your preferences. Start with a guided tour to familiarize yourself with a destination, then venture out on your own with newfound confidence.

And of course, travel insurance is non-negotiable. As we age, our healthcare needs may change, making insurance coverage more critical than ever. Take the time to understand your policy and ensure it adequately addresses your needs.

Finally, safety should always be a top priority. While solo travel is incredibly rewarding, it's essential to stay vigilant, especially as we grow older. Familiarize yourself with safety tips and precautions to ensure a smooth and enjoyable journey.

So, are you ready to embark on this incredible adventure? Embrace the freedom, the excitement, and the endless possibilities that solo travel in retirement has to offer. It's time to write the next chapter of your life—one unforgettable journey at a time.

Overcoming Common Obstacles and Fears Related to Travel

It's common to encounter obstacles and fears that might hold you back from fully enjoying your travel adventures. But the right strategies and mindset can help you overcome these hurdles and make your retirement travel dreams a reality!

Common obstacles and fears:

- **Safety concerns:** Many retirees worry about safety while traveling, especially in unfamiliar places or countries with different cultures.

- **Health and wellness:** Concerns about health issues, such as mobility limitations, medical emergencies, or simply feeling out of place in a new environment, can dampen the enthusiasm for travel.

- **Language barriers:** Not being able to communicate effectively due to language differences can make travel seem daunting and intimidating.

- **Loneliness:** Traveling alone might lead to feelings of loneliness or isolation, particularly for retirees who are used to companionship in their daily lives.

Strategies for overcoming obstacles:

- **Research safe destinations:** Take the time to thoroughly research destinations before you travel. Look for places that have a reputation for being safe for tourists, with low crime rates and good healthcare facilities. Websites like the U.S. Department of State's travel advisories and forums like TripAdvisor can provide valuable insights from other travelers.

- **Stay updated on health recommendations:** Keep yourself informed about health recommendations and requirements for your chosen destination. Check for any necessary vaccinations, travel restrictions, or health precautions you need to take before and during your trip. Always speak to your doctor before traveling.

- **Learn basic phrases:** While you don't need to become fluent in the local language, learning some basic phrases can go a long way in making you feel more comfortable and connected during your travels. Consider using language learning apps or taking online classes to familiarize yourself with essential phrases for communication.

- **Join travel groups or programs:** Traveling with a group or participating in organized travel programs can provide a sense of security and companionship. Look for travel groups specifically tailored to retirees or seniors, where you can connect with like-minded individuals and share experiences.

Remember, retirement is a time to have those new experiences and create lasting memories. Face those common obstacles with courage and preparation, and you can unlock the full potential of your retirement travels and start an unforgettable adventure around the globe!

Finding Meaning and Cultural Experiences Through Travel

While you are jumping on the travel bandwagon, why not immerse yourself in the culture and continue to learn about the world you live in? Here are some effective strategies to discover meaning and cultural experiences during your travels:

- **Immerse yourself in local culture:**
  - Take the time to learn about the customs, traditions, and history of the places you visit. Engage with locals by attending cultural events, festivals, and ceremonies. For example, in Japan, you might participate in a tea ceremony or learn the art of origami. If you are staying local, maybe you visit some great barbecue places in Texas and attend a rodeo!
  - Seek out authentic experiences such as homestays or cooking classes where you can interact with locals on a deeper level and gain insight into their way of life.

- **Interact with locals:**
  - Don't hesitate to strike up conversations with locals. You'll find that many people are eager to share their stories, traditions, and local recommendations. Whether it's chatting with a street vendor or joining a community group, these interactions can lead to meaningful connections and memorable experiences.
  - Consider volunteering opportunities or cultural exchange programs that allow you to work alongside locals and contribute to their communities. This not only fosters cultural

understanding but also provides a sense of fulfillment and purpose.

- **Participate in cultural activities:**
  - Explore the arts scene by visiting museums, galleries, and theaters. Attend performances of traditional music, dance, or theater to gain insight into the local culture's artistic expressions.
  - Take part in hands-on activities like traditional craft workshops or indigenous cultural experiences. For instance, in Peru, you might learn how to weave textiles or participate in a traditional Andean ceremony.

- **Support local communities through responsible tourism:**
  - Choose accommodations, restaurants, and tour operators that prioritize sustainability and responsible practices. Look for eco-friendly lodges, locally-owned guesthouses, and tour companies that support community-based tourism initiatives.
  - Be mindful of your environmental impact by minimizing waste, conserving resources, and respecting natural habitats. Consider participating in eco-tours or conservation projects that contribute to the preservation of local ecosystems.
  - Support local artisans and businesses by purchasing handmade crafts, locally-produced goods, and souvenirs that directly benefit the community. By investing in local economies, you're not only enriching your own travel experience but also making a positive impact on the lives of those you encounter.

Creating Lifelong Memories and Embracing New Horizons

We have covered an extensive amount of information about retirement and what this phase in your life could mean. What does it look like for you? How do you want to spend this time? Are you ready to start an amazing new chapter?

Embracing new experiences:

- **Stay curious:** Don't forget to cultivate a mindset of curiosity. Approach each day with an open mind and a willingness to explore the unknown.

- **Try something new:** Keep challenging yourself to step out of your comfort zone regularly. Whether it's learning a new hobby, trying a new cuisine, or traveling to a place you've never been, embracing new experiences keeps life vibrant and exciting.

- **Stay active:** Engage in physical activities that you enjoy. Whether it's hiking, dancing, or yoga, staying active not only benefits your physical health but also opens doors to new experiences and connections.

Making new friends:

- **Join clubs or groups:** Find those clubs or community groups that align with your interests. Look for that book club, a gardening group, or a volunteer organization, that provides an opportunities for you to meet like-minded people.

- **Stay socially connected:** Utilize social media platforms to reconnect with old friends and stay connected with family members. Try to attend social events and gatherings regularly to expand your social circle.

- **Be open-minded:** Don't forget to embrace diversity and be open to befriending people from different backgrounds and age groups. Every person has a unique story to share, and welcoming new friendships enriches your life in countless ways.

Creating meaningful memories:

- **Document your adventures:** Try keeping a journal, creating photo albums, or starting a blog to document your experiences and reflections. These tangible reminders of your journey will become cherished mementos over time.

- **Plan purposeful trips:** Travel to destinations that hold personal significance or offer cultural enrichment. Why not revisit a childhood home or explore a new country? Prioritize experiences that align with your passions and values.

- **Celebrate milestones:** Take time to acknowledge and celebrate milestones, both big and small. Acknowledge significant birthdays, an anniversary, or achieving a personal goal. Commemorating these moments creates lasting memories and reinforces a sense of accomplishment.

Remember, retirement is a chapter of life brimming with possibilities. When you start experiencing new things, forging meaningful connections, and creating lasting memories, you will gain fulfillment, growth, and joy. Grab the opportunity to see new things and make the most of this precious time in your life!

By discovering new things, you take a big step toward creating an enjoyable and lively retirement. As you think about the advice and tips given here, remember that retirement isn't just about getting to a goal; it's about welcoming the endless opportunities each day brings.

Traveling and seeking adventure in retirement is about expanding your horizons, igniting your sense of wonder, and creating lasting memories. Whether you're exploring far-flung corners of the globe or discovering hidden gems in your own backyard, each experience has the power to enrich your life in profound ways.

As you prepare to embark on your next adventure, do so with optimism, enthusiasm, and a spirit of adventure. Your journey awaits, and the world is yours to explore. Here's to a retirement filled with unforgettable experiences and endless happiness! Bon voyage, and may your travels be filled with laughter, discovery, and endless possibilities!

CONCLUSION

As we come to the end of our time together, I want to extend my sincere gratitude for joining me on this path toward a fulfilling retirement. Together, we've uncovered the nine essential habits that can lead to a retirement filled with joy, purpose, and contentment. Let's take a moment to reflect on the wisdom we've gained.

We started by getting ready for retirement. By preparing well, you've given yourself the tools to handle the ebbs and flows of this new phase in life. We've moved through different parts of retirement, accepting change and the new options it brings.

Central to our discussion is the importance of having a positive mindset, which helps you deal with life's changes in a strong and resilient way. We have also talked about the many advantages of finding new hobbies, taking care of your body, and building meaningful relationships with others.

Let's remember the importance to keep learning and growing throughout your life. Learning new things and following your passions makes your life full. Also, helping others through kindness, volunteering, and giving to charity not only helps them but also makes you feel fulfilled and purposeful.

And, of course, we got excited about travel and adventure. We spent time discovering the hidden benefits of planning and budgeting. It was great to realize the newfound freedom and exploration retirement offers.

As you close this book and reflect on the insights gained, remember this is not goodbye. I ask you to treat this book as a reference—a source of knowledge to return to whenever you seek inspiration or guidance. Don't hesitate to return to sections for refreshers when needed.

I want to leave you with this. You have dedicated decades of hard work and perseverance to your profession. As you start this next phase of your life, I encourage you to embrace the boundless opportunities that retirement affords. This is your time to rediscover the joys of life, to pursue passions long set aside, and to embark on new adventures with a spirit of enthusiasm, positivity, and curiosity. Retirement is a time to savor the simple pleasures of life, to bask in the beauty of each moment, and to cultivate a sense of gratitude for all that you have experienced and achieved. As a retiree, you have earned the right to live life on your own terms—to chart your own course and to pursue the passions and pursuits that bring you the greatest joy and fulfillment. So, as you step forward into retirement, do so with hope in your heart, confidence in your stride, and a steadfast belief in the abundant opportunities that await you.

In closing, if you found this book to be a valuable companion on your journey toward a happy retirement, I humbly ask for your review. Your words have the power to light the path for future retirees seeking guidance and support.

With warmest regards and best wishes for your continued happiness and fulfillment.

ABOUT THE AUTHOR

Sarah is a seasoned business leader with over three decades of experience spanning diverse industries and continents. Born in Gibraltar, she embarked on a global journey that led her from the UK to Australia, Japan, and she now resides in Dubai in the Middle East.

Her professional odyssey began in merchant banking before transitioning through fashion buying and multimedia events, ultimately finding her niche in the advertising space of creative and digital production. With a career dedicated to managing large cross-functional teams, Sarah understands the intricacies of cultivating positive work environments where individuals are valued for their contributions.

Beyond her professional life, Sarah is a certified Life and Retirement Coach, driven by her passion for empowering others to embrace authenticity and live boldly. Looking to her own future Sarah quickly became clear it's crucial we rethink what retirement means. Today, retirees are a vibrant, diverse bunch, spanning a spectrum of interests, passions, and energy levels and retirement is not a one-size-fits-all affair. And Sarah is dedicated to supporting this 'retirement' narrative rewrite.

Her focus is preparing to embrace the dawning of this new stage with freedom, fulfilment and happiness. Having a comfortable nest egg is essential and Sarah leaves this to the financial experts to provide guidance. Her focus is on, what good is that nest egg if you haven't considered how you will fill your days, once the alarm clock is retired too.

This journey led to Sarah's latest endeavor, *9 Habits of Happy Retirees*, where she hopes to provide guidance and support in embracing a new lifestyle of genuine happiness and fulfillment.

JOIN OUR MAILING LIST

Scan the QR code below to sign up to our Newsletter mailing list and receive your free bonus gift.

Our newsletters are full of valuable insights and helpful tips on retirement planning and lifestyle enhancement. We promise to deliver quality content that's both informative and inspiring, without overwhelming your inbox with unnecessary emails.

SCAN ME

REFERENCES

Aging changes in the bones - muscles - joints Information. (2023). Mount Sinai Health System. https://www.mountsinai.org/health-library/special-topic/aging-changes-in-the-bones-muscles-joints

Andrew Carnegie's story. (2019). Carnegie.org; Carnegie Corporation of New York. https://www.carnegie.org/interactives/foundersstory/

Breeding, B. (2020, September 21). Kindness matters: How volunteering can benefit seniors' health. *MyLifeSite.* https://mylifesite.net/blog/post/kindness-matters-how-volunteering-can-benefit-seniors-health/

Cook, S., Sladowski, P., Light, A., Bennett, S., & Hientz, M. (2013). *Volunteering and older adults.* Volunteer Canada. https://volunteer.ca/vdemo/EngagingVolunteers_DOCS/Volunteering_and_Older_Adults_Final_Report_2013.pdf

Crabtree, S. (2011, December 12). *U.S. seniors maintain happiness highs with less social time.* Gallup. https://news.gallup.com/poll/151457/seniors-maintain-happiness-highs-less-social-time.aspx

Five Common Misconceptions About Retirement. (2023, September 19). *Popular Blog.* https://blog.popular.com/en/five-common-misconceptions-about-retirement/

Healthy meal planning: Tips for older adults. (2021, November 23). National Institute on Aging. https://www.nia.nih.gov/health/healthy-eating-nutrition-and-diet/healthy-meal-planning-tips-older-adults

Hiles, C. (2024, March 25). *Senior citizens can go to college for free or cheap in all 50 states.* The Penny Hoarder. https://www.thepennyhoarder.com/save-money/free-college-courses-for-senior-citizens/

Himmer, R. (2024, February 29). *How to avoid the emotional challenges of retirement.* IG Wealth Management. https://www.ig.ca/en/insights/how-to-avoid-the-emotional-challenges-of-retirement

How much physical activity do older adults need? (2023, April 13). Centers for Disease Control and Prevention. https://www.cdc.gov/physicalactivity/basics/older_adults/index.htm

Hughes, D. (2021, February 28). *Why you still need time management after you retire.* Retire Fabulously. https://retirefabulously.com/still-need-time-management-retire/

The importance of feeling connected. (2022, January 28). *Homestead Village.* https://www.homesteadvillage.org/blog/the-importance-of-feeling-connected/

Lagemann, J. (2022, September 30). *11 meaningful ways older adults can volunteer right now.* Forbes Health. https://www.forbes.com/health/healthy-aging/volunteer-opportunities-for-older-adults/

Lee, L. O., James, P., Zevon, E. S., Kim, E. S., Trudel-Fitzgerald, C., Spiro, A., Grodstein, F., & Kubzansky, L. D. (2019). Optimism is associated with exceptional longevity in 2 epidemiologic cohorts of men and women. *Proceedings of the National Academy of Sciences, 116*(37), 18357–18362. https://doi.org/10.1073/pnas.1900712116

Loneliness and social isolation linked to serious health conditions. (2021, April 29). Centers for Disease Control and Prevention. https://www.cdc.gov/aging/publications/features/lonely-older-adults.html

Mayer, B. A. (2021, October 20). Your sleep needs change as you age: Here's what you need to know. *Healthline.* https://www.healthline.com/health/healthy-sleep/your-sleep-needs-change-as-you-age-heres-what-you-need-to-know

Murray, K. O., Mahoney, S. A., Venkatasubramanian, R., Seals, D. R., & Clayton, Z. S. (2023). Aging, aerobic exercise, and cardiovascular health: Barriers, alternative strategies and future directions. *Experimental Gerontology, 173,* 112105. https://doi.org/10.1016/j.exger.2023.112105

Never too late: Exercise helps late starters. (2011, March 1). Harvard Health. https://www.health.harvard.edu/mens-health/never-too-late-exercise-helps-late-starters

Piolatto, M., Bianchi, F., Rota, M., Marengoni, A., Akbaritabar, A., & Squazzoni, F. (2022). The effect of social relationships on cognitive decline in older adults: an updated systematic review and meta-analysis of longitudinal cohort studies. *BMC Public Health*, *22*(1). https://doi.org/10.1186/s12889-022-12567-5

Prvulovic, T. (2021, September 13). *Social life after retirement - 22 ways to improve it.* Second Wind Movement. https://secondwindmovement.com/social-life-after-retirement/

Prvulovic, T. (2022, July 11). *The 5 emotional stages of retirement: How to adjust.* Second Wind Movement. https://secondwindmovement.com/retirement-stages/

Public Health Agency of Canada. (2021, July 14). *Aging and chronic diseases: A profile of Canadian seniors.* Www.canada.ca. https://www.canada.ca/en/public-health/services/publications/diseases-conditions/aging-chronic-diseases-profile-canadian-seniors-report.html

Reid, S. (2024, February 5). *Gratitude: The benefits and how to practice it* . Https://Www.helpguide.org. https://www.helpguide.org/articles/mental-health/gratitude.htm#:~:text=Acknowledging%20gratitude%20also%20decreases%20stress

Retirement confidence survey. (2022). In *Greenwald Research* (pp. 3–9). https://www.ebri.org/docs/default-source/rcs/2022-rcs/2022-rcs-summary-report.pdf

Robinson, L., Segal, J., & Smith, M. (2018, November 2). *The mental health benefits of exercise* . Https://Www.helpguide.org. https://www.helpguide.org/articles/healthy-living/the-mental-health-benefits-of-exercise.htm#:~:text=Regular%20exercise%20can%20have%20a

The Rockefellers: A legacy of giving. (2017). Rockefeller Philanthropy Advisors. https://www.rockpa.org/guide/rockefellers-legacy-giving/

Rosenberg, R. (2024, March 25). *Want to travel the world in retirement? Here's how.* Investopedia. https://www.investopedia.com/traveling-during-retirement-7564945#:~:text=%E2%80%9CRetirees%20spend%2C%20on%20average%2C

Royal, J. R. (2023, November 22). *How to gain confidence in your retirement strategy: 5 areas you must address.* Bankrate. https://www.bankrate.com/retirement/confidence-retirement-strategy/#:~:text=%E2%80%9CConnecting%20with%20your%20advisor%20or

Schroeder, J. (2020, August 30). *7 surprisingly valuable assets for a happy retirement.* Kiplinger. https://www.kiplinger.com/retirement/happy-retirement/601160/7-surprisingly-valuable-assets-for-a-happy-retirement

Senior Experts. (2022, August 22). Retirement expectations influence how retirees adjust to the change in their lives. *LinkedIn.* https://www.linkedin.com/pulse/retirement-expectations-influence-how-retirees-adjust-change-/

The 7 best retirement hobbies for creative types. (2023, April 4). Www.vistaspringsliving.com. https://www.vistaspringsliving.com/blog/the-7-best-retirement-hobbies-for-creative-types

Sites, S. (2023, December 1). *10 strategies to build resilience after retirement.* Discovery Village. https://www.discoveryvillages.com/senior-living-blog/10-strategies-to-build-resilience-after-retirement/#:~:text=Pursuing%20Lifelong%20Learning

Statistics Canada. (2015, July 17). *Health Reports: Community belonging and self-perceived health, findings.* Www150.Statcan.gc.ca. https://www150.statcan.gc.ca/n1/pub/82-003-x/2008002/article/10552/5202483-eng.htm

Sullivan Killroy, D. (2014, September 8). *Exercise plan for seniors.* Healthline; Healthline Media. https://www.healthline.com/health/everyday-fitness/senior-workouts

Technology for seniors : Staying connected in the digital age . (2023, December 21). Visavie. https://visavie.com/en/technology-for-seniors-staying-connected-in-the-digital-age

Thoreau, H.D. (n.d.). *Henry David Thoreau quotes.* Goodreads. https://www.goodreads.com/quotes/8105541-go-confidently-in-the-direction-of-your-dreams-live-the

Waugh, J. (2023, May 22). *Solo travel in retirement: Relaunch life with surprising tips.* Solo Traveler. https://solotravelerworld.com/solo-travel-in-retirement-relaunch-life-with-surprising-tips/

What are the five stages of retirement? (2023, February 6). Caring Places Management. https://www.caringplaces.com/what-are-the-five-stages-of-retirement/

Wu, Y.-T., Luben, R., & Jones, A. (2017). Dog ownership supports the maintenance of physical activity during poor weather in older English adults: cross-sectional results from the EPIC Norfolk cohort. *Journal of Epidemiology and Community Health, 71*(9), 905–911. https://doi.org/10.1136/jech-2017-208987

Made in the USA
Columbia, SC
29 November 2024

47871457R00081